Coding and Reimbursement for Hospital Inpatient Services

SECOND EDITION

Karen S. Scott, MEd, RHIA, CCS-P, CPC

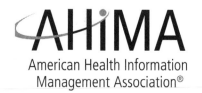

American Health Information
Management Association®

The contents of this workbook are based on the *ICD-9-CM* updates of October 1, 2007, through September 30, 2008; fiscal year 2008 short-term acute care hospitals, long-term acute care hospitals, and inpatient rehabilitation facilities; and rate year 2008 for inpatient psychiatric facilities.

This book contains material originally published as *Coding for Prospective Payment*, by Rita K. Finnegan, and *Applying Inpatient Coding Skills under Prospective Payment, 2004 edition*, by Vickie L. Rogers and Ann M. Zeisset.

ISBN 1-58426-198-6
ISBN-13 978-1-58426-198-8
Product No. AC206208

Claire Blondeau, MBA, Senior Editor
Katherine Greenock, Assistant Editor
Carol Spencer, RHIA, Manager, Professional Practice Resources
Melissa Ulbricht, Editorial/Production Coordinator
Ken Zielske, Director of Publications

American Health Information Management Association
233 North Michigan Avenue, 21st Floor
Chicago, Illinois 60601-5800
http://ahima.org

Contents

About the Author v

Preface vii

Note to Educators ix

Part I   Reimbursement Systems for Inpatient Services

Chapter 1   Introduction to Hospital Inpatient Services 3

Chapter 2   Reimbursement Methodologies for Inpatient Services 15

Chapter 3   Structure and Organization of the Medicare Inpatient
             Acute Care Prospective Payment System 29

Chapter 4   Structure and Organization of Other Medicare Inpatient
             Prospective Payment Systems 47

Part II   Coding for Inpatient Services

Chapter 5   Diagnostic and Procedural Coding for Inpatient Services. 61

Chapter 6   Coding and DRG Assignment 73

**Part III   Processes Related to Coding and Reimbursement
             for Inpatient Services**

Chapter 7   Data Quality Management. 93

Chapter 8   Coding Compliance 101

Chapter 9   The Health Record Auditing Process. 115

Exercises. 125

Case Studies. 135

Appendix A   AHIMA Code of Ethics 149

Appendix B   AHIMA Practice Brief:
                  Developing a Coding Compliance Policy Document 159

Appendix C   AHIMA Practice Brief: Developing a Physician Query Process. 165

Appendix D   Data Quality: The Impact on Healthcare and HIM 175

Appendix E   AHIMA Practice Brief: Managing and Improving Data Quality 181

Appendix F   Developing an Effective Compliance Audit Process 187

Appendix G   Sample Audit Worksheets, Forms, and Tools. 201

Abbreviations 213

Annotated Bibliography 219

References 221

Index 225

CD-ROM Contents

Exercises

Case Studies

Sample Audit Worksheets, Forms, and Tools

References with Live Web Links

About the Author

Karen S. Scott, MEd, RHIA, CCS-P, CPC, is a registered health information administrator (RHIA) with more than 20 years' experience in the healthcare field. She has earned the certified coding specialist-physician based (CCS-P) credential from AHIMA, as well as the certified professional coder (CPC) credential from the American Academy of Professional Coders (AAPC).

Scott is owner of Karen Scott Seminars and Consulting. She has been an educator for many years and has taught in health information management (HIM) programs at the University of Tennessee Health Science Center and Arkansas Tech University. She holds a BS in HIM and an MEd in instructional technology from Arkansas Tech University in Russellville. She is past president of both the Tennessee and Arkansas HIM associations and is past chair of the AHIMA Council on Certification. The Tennessee Health Information Management Association (THIMA) awarded Scott its Distinguished Member Award in 2005.

Scott teaches seminars on coding, reimbursement, medical terminology, and management throughout the country. She has published numerous articles on various healthcare topics and has written several chapters in other HIM and coding textbooks.

Preface

Coding and Reimbursement for Hospital Inpatient Services, Second Edition was written for coding practitioners who have previous knowledge of, and coding experience with, the *International Classification of Diseases, 9th Revision, Clinical Modification* (ICD-9-CM). It includes and expands on the material previously published by AHIMA in the book, *Applying Inpatient Coding Skills under Prospective Payment, 2004 edition,* by Vickie L. Rogers and Ann M. Zeisset.

The reimbursement material in this book is specific to hospital inpatient settings, that is, to hospitals paid under Medicare prospective payment systems:

- The inpatient prospective payment system (IPPS)

- The long-term care hospital prospective payment system (LTCH-PPS)

- The inpatient rehabilitation facilities prospective payment system (IRF-PPS)

- The inpatient psychiatric facility prospective payment system (IPF-PPS)

Part I, Reimbursement Systems for Inpatient Services, contains chapters 1 through 4, which provide the reader with a fundamental understanding of reimbursement methodologies under Medicare prospective payment. Chapter 1 provides an introduction to hospital inpatient services and discusses the different types of services provided in various inpatient settings. Chapter 2 presents an in-depth overview of inpatient reimbursement methodologies, focusing on the array of payment systems used to reimburse hospitals for inpatient services and discussing some of the most common payers in the U.S. health system. Chapter 3 contains a detailed discussion of the structure and organization of Medicare prospective payment for inpatient acute care, which centers on the DRG reimbursement system. Chapter 4 explains the structure and organization of other Medicare inpatient prospective payment systems, including the LTCH-PPS, IRF-PPS, and IPF-PPS, with their various patient assignment and payment classifications.

Part II, Coding for Inpatient Services, contains two chapters that deal with the technical and professional aspects of coding practice. Chapter 5 addresses both diagnostic and procedural coding for inpatient services and includes information on the ICD-9-CM Official Guidelines for Coding and Reporting, coding ethics, and billing processes, among other subjects. Chapter 6 discusses coding and DRG assignment, and covers topics such as coding with incomplete information, understanding case mix and case-mix management, understanding paired DRGs and benchmarks, and using physician query forms.

Part III, Processes Related to Coding and Reimbursement for Inpatient Services, contains chapters 7, 8, and 9, which introduce the reader to data quality management, coding compliance, and health record auditing.

The chapters are supplemented by exercises, case studies, and appendices, which include AHIMA's Standards for Ethical Coding and Code of Ethics, an annotated bibliography of coding references, the AHIMA practice brief on developing a coding compliance policy document, and sample audit forms and tools.

Note to Educators

An answer key for all exercises included in this book is available in online format from the individual book pages in the AHIMA Bookstore and through the Assembly on Education (AOE) Community of Practice (CoP) under Community Resources/Instructor Materials. Instructors who are AHIMA members can sign up for this private community by clicking on the help icon on the CoP home page and requesting additional information on becoming an AOE CoP member. An instructor who is not an AHIMA member or an AHIMA member who is not an instructor may contact the publisher at publications@ahima.org. The instructor materials are not available to students enrolled in college or university programs.

Use of different versions of coding books with this resource will require attention to the code changes after the effective date. Revised answer keys will be created that are consistent with coding changes for the upcoming year soon after the effective date of the new codes. All answer keys are available to instructors in online format from the individual book page in the AHIMA Bookstore (http://imis.ahima.org/orders) and also are posted on the AOE CoP Web site. Instructors who are AHIMA members can sign up for this private community by clicking on the help icon on the CoP home page and requesting additional information on becoming an AOE CoP member. An instructor who is not an AHIMA member or a member who is not an instructor may contact the publisher at publications@ahima.org.

Part I

Reimbursement Systems for Inpatient Services

Chapter 1

Introduction to Hospital Inpatient Services

An inpatient is defined as "A person who has been admitted at least overnight to a hospital or other health facility for the purpose of receiving diagnostic treatment or other health services" (Southeast Tennessee Legal Services n.d.).

However, there are times when patients are formally admitted to the hospital but, for whatever reason, are either discharged or transferred without actually staying overnight. An inpatient admission begins with the formal acceptance by a hospital of a patient who is to receive healthcare while receiving room, board, and continuous nursing services (CMS 2006a). It is the responsibility of the admitting physician to determine the appropriateness of admission to the hospital, but the admission process is monitored by hospital staff to ensure that documentation and clinical information support the need for hospital admission.

The physician typically uses a 24-hour period as a benchmark; that is, he or she orders inpatient admission for patients who are expected to need hospital care for 24 hours or more and treat other patients on an outpatient basis. However, the decision to admit a patient is a complex medical judgment that can be made only after the physician has considered a number of factors, including the patient's medical history and current medical needs, the types of facilities available to inpatients and to outpatients, the hospital's bylaws and admissions policies, and the relative appropriateness of treatment in each setting. Factors to be considered when making the decision to admit include such things as:

- The severity of the signs and symptoms exhibited by the patient

- The medical predictability of something adverse happening to the patient

- The need for diagnostic studies that appropriately are outpatient services (that is, their performance does not ordinarily require the patient to remain at the hospital for 24 hours or more) to assist in assessing whether the patient should be admitted

- The availability of diagnostic procedures at the time when and at the location where the patient presents

This chapter discusses the different services provided in the inpatient setting. The most familiar type of inpatient service is acute care, short-term hospitalization. Most patients in this setting are either medical or surgical patients.

Medical Services

Medical services are those services provided to patients who do not require surgery to correct or enhance body functions. These services may be subdivided according to hospital needs into specific services, such as internal medicine and pediatrics. Common service divisions are as follows:

- *Internal medicine:* Nonsurgical treatment for adults

- *Pediatrics:* Nonsurgical treatment for children

- *Obstetrics/gynecology:* Diagnosis and treatment for female reproductive system conditions including pregnancy-related conditions

- *Cardiology:* Diagnosis and treatment of diseases of the heart and circulatory system

Some services are divided based on body system or organs treated both surgically and medically, such as:

- *Orthopedics:* Treatment of bones and joints

- *Urology:* Treatment of the urinary system

- *Gastroenterology:* Diagnosis and treatment of disorders of the digestive tract

- *Pulmonary medicine:* Diagnosis and treatment of disorders of the respiratory system

- *Neurology:* Treatment of conditions of the nerves

Surgical Services

Surgery is defined as "a procedure to remove or repair a part of the body or to find out whether disease is present" (University of Texas 2008). General surgery consists of surgeries to correct conditions in various body systems. Traditionally, general surgeons perform surgeries such as cholecystectomies, mastectomies, hernia repairs, and gastric bypass procedures.

Surgical services may be subdivided based on the body system that is treated, such as:

- *Cardiothoracic surgery:* This service refers to the surgical treatment of the heart and other conditions of the vascular system.

- *Bariatric surgery:* This specialty focuses on weight reduction surgery for morbidly obese patients through the use of techniques such as gastric bypass and gastric banding procedures.

- *Plastic surgery:* According to the American Society of Plastic Surgeons, plastic surgery consists of both cosmetic and reconstructive surgery.

  Cosmetic surgery is performed to reshape normal structures of the body in order to improve the patient's appearance and self-esteem. Cosmetic surgery is usually not covered by health insurance because it is elective. Reconstructive surgery is performed on abnormal structures of the body, caused by congenital defects, developmental abnormalities, trauma, infection, tumors or disease. It is generally performed to improve functions, but may also be done to approximate a normal appearance. Reconstructive surgery is generally covered by most health insurance policies, although coverage for specific procedures and levels of coverage may vary greatly (ASPS 2008).

- *Neurosurgery:* This is the surgical treatment of diseases of the nervous system.

- *Oral and maxillofacial surgery:* This consists of surgical treatment of diseases of the mouth and facial region of the body. This sometimes includes reconstruction surgery to the face and jaw area.

- *Transplant surgery:* This deals with the transplant of organs such as kidney, liver, heart, and lungs. Transplant surgeons and their staff deal with pre- and postoperative treatment of transplant patients, including monitoring for organ rejection.

The Uniform Hospital Data Discharge Set (UHDDS) differentiates between a significant and nonsignificant procedure. A significant procedure is one that is:

- Surgical in nature

- Carries a procedural risk

- Carries an aesthetic risk

- Requires specialized training

Rehabilitation Services

Rehabilitation services are provided to patients who have had a previous illness or injury that limits their physical or mental capabilities. These services may be provided as part of the patient's acute care hospitalization or given in an extended care facility. Rehabilitation hospitals or hospital units focus on restoring the patient's functions to the greatest extent possible. Inpatient rehabilitation facilities are known as IRFs.

According to Medicare regulations, inpatient rehabilitation is covered only when the service is considered to be reasonable and medically necessary based on the individual patient's needs.

Preadmission screening is required to help make this determination prior to admission to an IRF. Much of the information that is used in this determination is taken from the documentation in the acute care patient medical record. Examples of the appropriate use of rehabilitation services provided include:

- *After an inpatient hospital stay for rehabilitation care that resulted in little improvement in the patient's condition:* For example, an individual who undergoes surgery for severe contractures as a result of arthritis may require a reassessment of his or her rehabilitation potential in light of the surgery.

- *After an inpatient stay for cerebral vascular accident (CVA) with residual impairments:* The fact that an individual has some degree of mental impairment is not per se a basis for concluding that a multidisciplinary team evaluation is not warranted. Many individuals who have had CVAs have both mental and physical impairments. The mental impairment often results in a limited attention span and reduced comprehension with a resultant problem in communication. With an intensive rehabilitation program, it is sometimes possible to correct or significantly alleviate both the mental and physical problems.

- *After an inpatient admission for an acute traumatic or infectious process, such as a hip fracture, with residual need for rehabilitation:* Absent other complicating medical problems, the type of rehabilitation program normally required by a patient with a fractured hip during or after the non-weight-bearing period or a patient with a healed ankle fracture does not require an inpatient hospital stay for rehabilitation care. Accordingly, an inpatient assessment is not warranted in such cases. On the other hand, an individual who has had a CVA that has left him or her significantly dependent in the activities of daily living (even after physical therapy in a different setting) might be a good candidate for a more extensive inpatient assessment if the patient has potential for rehabilitation and his or her needs are not primarily of a custodial nature (CMS 2007a).

Common criteria used to establish the need for inpatient rehabilitation services include the need for round-the-clock medical supervision and nursing care and approximately three hours of rehabilitation care per day at least five days per week. It must be established that the patient can make significant improvements in recovery through rehabilitation services.

Psychiatric Services

Jonas (1998, 53) defines psychiatric services as "diagnosis and therapy for people of all ages with psychological and emotional problems, using counseling, pharmaceutical, and other interventions." Inpatient psychiatric facilities (IPFs) may be independent or freestanding facilities or may consist of a unit within an acute care facility.

Medicare reimburses facilities for inpatient psychiatric hospital services only for "active treatment" that can reasonably be expected to improve the patient's condition. To ensure that the services provided meet this definition, the physician has to certify that the patient can benefit from inpatient psychiatric treatment. Medicare has established three criteria that must be addressed in the patient's medical documentation:

1. *Individualized treatment or diagnostic plan:* The services must be provided in accordance with an individualized program of treatment or diagnosis developed by a physician in conjunction with staff members of appropriate other disciplines on the basis of a thorough evaluation of the patient's restorative needs and potentialities. Thus, an isolated service such as a single session with a psychiatrist or a routine laboratory test not furnished under a planned program of therapy or diagnosis would not constitute active treatment, even though the service was therapeutic or diagnostic in nature.

   The plan of treatment must be recorded in the patient's medical record in accordance with section 405.l037(a)(8) of the regulations on Conditions of Participation for Hospitals.

2. *Services expected to improve the condition or for purpose of diagnosis:* The service must reasonably be expected to improve the patient's condition or must be for the purpose of diagnostic study. It is not necessary that a course of therapy have as its goal the restoration of the patient to a level that would permit discharge from the institution, although the treatment must, at a minimum, be designed to both reduce or control the patient's psychotic or neurotic symptoms that necessitated hospitalization *and* improve the patient's level of functioning.

   The kinds of services that meet the above requirements would include not only psychotherapy, drug therapy, and shock therapy, but also such adjunctive therapies as occupational therapy, recreational therapy, and milieu therapy, provided the adjunctive therapeutic services are expected to result in improvement (as defined above) in the patient's condition. If, however, the only activities prescribed for the patient are primarily diversional in nature (that is, to provide some social or recreational outlet for the patient), such services would not be regarded as treatment to improve the patient's condition. In many large hospitals, these adjunctive services are present and part of the life experience of every patient. In a case where milieu therapy (or one of the other adjunctive therapies) is involved, it is particularly important that this therapy be a planned program for the particular patient and not one in which life in the hospital is designated as milieu therapy.

3. *Services supervised and evaluated by a physician:* Physician participation in the services is an essential ingredient of active treatment. The services of qualified individuals other than physicians, such as social workers, occupational therapists, group therapists, attendants, and so forth, must be prescribed and directed by a physician to meet the specific psychiatric needs of the individual. In short, the physician must serve as a source of information and guidance for all members of the therapeutic team who work directly with the patient in various roles. It is the responsibility of the physician to periodically evaluate the therapeutic program and determine the extent to which treatment goals are being realized and whether changes in direction or emphasis are needed. Such evaluation should be made on the basis of periodic consultations and conferences with therapists, reviews of the patient's medical record, and regularly scheduled patient interviews, at least once a week (CMS 2007a).

Ancillary Services

Ancillary services typically included in an inpatient admission include nursing services, radiology, laboratory, physical and occupational therapy, respiratory therapy, speech therapy, medical social services, and case management services, in addition to other diagnostic and therapeutic services.

Nursing services

Nursing services are integral to the hospital admission. Nurses are the inpatient's primary caregivers, providing services as diverse as capturing vital signs, giving medications, and ensuring that the patient's needs are met. Nursing documentation assists physicians and other providers in assessing the patient's response to therapy and establishes a plan of action for future care.

Radiology Services

Radiology services in the hospital setting include both diagnostic and therapeutic services. Services such as computed tomography (CT) scan, magnetic resonance imaging (MRI), and ultrasound are commonly used to facilitate diagnosis of medical conditions. Nuclear medicine and interventional cardiology procedures may be used as either diagnostic or therapeutic treatment for diseases such as cancer and heart conditions.

Laboratory Services

Medicare defines a clinical laboratory as a "laboratory where microbiological, serological, chemical, hematological, radiobioassay, cytological, immunohematological, or pathological examinations are performed on materials derived from the human body, to provide information for the diagnosis, prevention, or treatment of a disease or assessment of a medical condition"

(CMS 2007a). A hospital medical laboratory is under the direction of a pathologist but is typically managed by medical technologists. Computer technology advances aid the medical technologists in performing a variety of laboratory tests designed to help with the diagnosis and evaluation of treatment methodology. Documentation of laboratory test results serves as further clinical proof of the existence of disease or can be used to determine that a patient does not have certain medical conditions.

Physical Therapy Services

Physical therapy is defined as (University of Tennessee 2007):

> . . . the examination, evaluation, intervention, and prevention of physical disability, movement dysfunction and pain resulting from injury, disease, disability, or other health-related conditions. Physical therapy includes:
>
> 1. The performance and interpretation of tests and measurements to assess pathophysiological, pathomechanical, electrophysiological, ergonomic, and developmental deficits of bodily systems to determine diagnosis, intervention, prognosis, and prevention
> 2. The planning, administration, and modification of therapeutic interventions that focus on posture, locomotion, strength, endurance, cardiopulmonary function, balance, coordination, joint mobility, flexibility, pain, healing and repair, and functional abilities in daily living skills, including work
> 3. The provision of consultative, educational, research, and other advisory services

Medicare has set up very specific payment rules to determine whether the prescribed physical therapy services are medically necessary. This means that the services must be considered by standards of care to be effective treatment for the condition and that the treatment will cause the patient's condition to improve. Documentation by the physical therapy providers should be sufficient to prove medical necessity and to justify all treatment modalities as well as to show the amount of time and level of supervision required for the services rendered.

Occupational Therapy Services

Occupational therapy is used to help to improve functions of the body that have been damaged due to injury or illness. The goal of occupational therapy is to improve the patient's ability to carry on with activities of daily living, such as dressing, cooking, or adapting to working conditions. According to Medicare, these services may include:

- The evaluation (and reevaluation as required) of a patient's level of function by administering diagnostic and prognostic tests

- The selection and teaching of task-oriented therapeutic activities designed to restore physical function—for example, use of woodworking activities on an inclined table to restore shoulder, elbow, and wrist range of motion lost as a result of burns

- The planning, implementing, and supervising of individualized therapeutic activity programs as part of an overall "active treatment" program for a patient with a diagnosed psychiatric illness—for example, sewing activities that require following a pattern to reduce confusion and restore reality orientation in a schizophrenic patient

- The planning and implementing of therapeutic tasks and activities to restore sensory-integrative function—for example, providing motor and tactile activities to increase sensory input and improve response for a stroke patient with functional loss resulting in a distorted body image

- The teaching of compensatory technique to improve the level of independence in activities of daily living

- The designing, fabricating, and fitting of orthotic and self-help devices—for example, making a hand splint for a patient with rheumatoid arthritis to maintain the hand in a functional position or constructing a device that would enable an individual to hold a utensil and feed himself or herself independently

Respiratory Therapy Services

Respiratory therapy, or respiratory care, provides both diagnostic and therapeutic services designed to evaluate and treat conditions associated with the patient's respiratory system. Respiratory therapy professionals also participate in the care of the critically ill patient by monitoring life-sustaining equipment such as mechanical ventilators.

According to Medicare's definitions, respiratory therapy services include services such as:

- The application of techniques for support of oxygenation and ventilation in the acutely ill patient. These techniques include, but are not limited to:

  —Establishment and maintenance of artificial airways

  —Ventilator therapy and other means of airway pressure manipulation

  —Precise delivery of oxygen concentration

  —Techniques to aid removal of secretions from the pulmonary tree

- The therapeutic use and monitoring of medical gases (especially oxygen), bland and pharmacologically active mists and aerosols, and such equipment as resuscitators and ventilators

- Bronchial hygiene therapy, including deep breathing and coughing exercises, intermittent positive pressure breathing (IPPB), postural drainage, chest percussion and vibration, and nasotracheal suctioning

- Diagnostic tests for evaluation by a physician, such as pulmonary function tests, spirometry, and blood gas analyses

- Pulmonary rehabilitation techniques, which include:

  —Exercise conditioning

  —Breathing retraining

  —Patient education regarding the management of the patient's respiratory problems

- Periodic assessment and monitoring of the acute and chronically ill patients for indications for, and the effectiveness of, respiratory therapy services (CMS 2007a).

Speech Therapy Services

Speech pathology services are those services necessary for the diagnosis and treatment of conditions regarding language, speech, and the voice. Most insurance companies reimburse only for services directly related to the treatment of disorders that hinder the patient's ability to communicate or for those conditions that impair the swallowing function.

Medical Social Services

Social services are designed to allow for assessment of an individual's emotional and social conditions to determine an appropriate plan of care. This may include evaluation of the individual's capability for self-care as well as the amount and type of care needed to assist the patient with recovery. In the hospital setting, social services are usually involved in discharge planning. This can entail nursing home placement or other types of home services that patients may require after discharge from the hospital.

Case Management Services

Case management in hospital and other healthcare systems is a collaborative practice model including patients, nurses, social workers, physicians, other practitioners, caregivers, and the community. The case management process encompasses communication and facilitates care along a continuum through effective resource coordination.

The goals of case management include the achievement of optimal health, access to care, and appropriate utilization of resources, balanced with the patient's right to self-determination. Among their many services to patients, case managers engage in the following activities:

- Working directly with patients and their families to provide information and emotional support

- Helping develop care plans

- Serving as the patient's advocate

- Coordinating medical care among different disciplines and specialties

- Helping patients establish their long- and short-term health goals

- Helping patients and families sort through and prioritize information needed to make decisions

- Helping with aftercare planning to foresee possible needs and coordinate referrals for services and equipment

- Working with insurance providers to ensure maximum coverage of services

Inpatient Accommodations

Most inpatient facilities offer various types of accommodations, including private and semi-private rooms, as well as specialty units such as intensive care and newborn nurseries. As new hospitals are being constructed and existing hospitals renovated, private rooms have become more standard.

Medicare, for example, allows a hospital to charge the patient an additional amount for a private room if the hospital has both private and semiprivate rooms available, as long as the private room is not medically necessary and if the patient has requested a private room and been notified of the additional charge.

Some common medically necessary reasons for private rooms include (CMS 2007a):

- *Need for isolation:* A private room is medically necessary in cases in which isolation of a beneficiary is required to avoid jeopardizing his or her health or recovery or that of other patients who are likely to be alarmed or disturbed by the beneficiary's symptoms or treatment or subjected to infection by the beneficiary's communicable disease. The private room must be ordered by the physician.

- *Admission required and only private rooms available:* A private room is considered to be medically necessary even though the beneficiary's condition does not require isolation if he or she needs immediate hospitalization (that is, his or her medical condition is such that hospitalization cannot be deferred) and the hospital has no semiprivate or ward accommodations available at the time of admission.

- *All-private room providers:* If the patient is admitted to a provider that has only private accommodations and no semiprivate or ward accommodations, medical necessity will be deemed to exist for the accommodations furnished. Beneficiaries may not be subjected to an extra charge for a private room in an all-private room provider.

Special Units

Special units for inpatients are equipped and staffed to provide specialized care that is focused on the specific needs of different patient populations. Among these special units are those for intensive care, coronary care, neonatal intensive care, nursery, and recuperative care.

Intensive Care

The intensive care unit (ICU) or critical care unit (CCU) is designed for the care-intensive patient who has sustained life-threatening illnesses or injury. It may consist of a wardlike atmosphere with multiple patients in a large room, or the patient areas may be divided into individual rooms. Patients in this unit receive intensive monitoring of vital signs and organ functioning by specially trained nursing professionals. Some facilities have special subdivisions of their ICUs to care for specific types of patients, such as coronary care, trauma care, or neonatal intensive care units.

Coronary Care

The coronary care unit may be included in the hospital's intensive care area or may be a distinct unit. Patients treated in the coronary care unit have heart-related conditions and require intensive cardiac monitoring. Patients recovering from open-heart surgery, such as a coronary artery bypass graft (CABG), may be placed in either the coronary care or a special postsurgical ICU.

Neonatal Intensive Care Unit

The neonatal intensive care unit (NICU) is a specially designed nursery. Premature and critically ill newborns frequently require long and resource-intensive medical evaluation and treatment. Because these babies may require a great deal of medical care during and after their recovery, staff in a typical NICU include specially trained nurses and neonatologists, social services representatives, and discharge planning personnel. Hospitals may have several levels of neonatal units, including one that specializes in babies recovering from surgery.

Nursery

The nursery is a unit designed to care for newborn babies who do not require the additional services provided in the NICU. Many facilities have a birthing center that allows for care of the mother and baby together, but separate newborn nurseries are still available to care for the healthy newborn for the first few days of life.

Recuperative Care/Swing Bed

Patients in small, rural hospitals may require short-term skilled nursing care following their acute care hospitalization. These facilities are allowed to use beds for acute care and to provide the skilled care as well. Because the hospital beds can be used as both acute care and skilled care beds, as needed, the term *swing bed* has been utilized. Under these regulations, a patient who meets criteria for skilled care may be discharged from acute care and admitted into swing bed care without physically changing beds. Because this is a discharge from one type of service to another, the physician and staff complete two separate sets of documentation, including a discharge summary from acute care and one from swing bed care.

In larger facilities, a patient needing skilled care would be discharged to a recuperative care patient unit in the hospital.

Types of Hospitals

Acute care hospitals designated as for-profit or not-for-profit healthcare systems are differentiated on the basis of ownership status. Other types of hospitals, such as Veterans Affairs (VA) healthcare facilities, short-term care acute hospitals, long-term acute care, children's hospitals, and critical access hospitals (CAHs), provide care for a specific population, duration, or locality and may operate under a unique reimbursement system.

For-Profit Hospitals

For-profit hospitals are usually owned by corporations whose shareholders own a portion of the business. There are several large for-profit hospital corporations in the United States.

Not-for-profit Hospitals

Not-for-profit hospitals are typically governed by a board of trustees or directors and do not have shareholders. The term *not for profit* is somewhat misleading in that not-for-profit hospitals are allowed to make a profit but do not have shareholders with expectations of specific profits.

Most not-for-profit hospitals are considered to be public hospitals and are owned by a church, a community organization, or a government agency such as a county. In a county-owned facility, the board of trustees/directors is usually chaired by the county judge or mayor and the board is made up of elected or appointed members of the community.

Veterans Hospitals

The federal government established VA hospitals in 1930 to care for wounded soldiers returning from war. According to the Department of Veterans Affairs, more than seven million veterans were enrolled in the VA healthcare system in 2004. There are approximately 157 medical centers across the country with more than 1,300 sites of care, including outpatient clinics, nursing homes, home healthcare, and rehabilitation treatment programs. Veterans with service-connected injuries or disabilities are treated at no cost to them. Other veterans may receive treatment at VA hospitals, but their insurance company can be billed for treatment of non–service-connected conditions. VA hospitals are commonly located in medical centers where they serve as teaching sites for medical students, residents, and other healthcare professionals.

Short-Term Acute Care Hospitals

Short-term acute care hospitals generally provide services to patients recovering from surgery or being treated for acute illnesses and injuries. Short-term care is usually considered to be less than thirty days.

Long-Term Acute Care Hospitals

Medicare defines long-term acute care hospitals (LTCHs) as hospitals that "have an average inpatient length of stay greater than 25 days. These hospitals typically provide extended medical and rehabilitative care for patients who are clinically complex and may suffer from multiple acute or chronic conditions. Services may include comprehensive rehabilitation, respiratory therapy, cancer treatment, head trauma treatment and pain management" (CMS 2004a).

Critical Access Hospitals

Medicare has determined that some hospitals are exempt from prospective payment systems (PPSs). As part of the Balanced Budget Act of 1997, the government established the Medicare Rural Hospital Flexibility Program, which enabled some hospitals to be designated as Critical Access Hospitals. A critical access hospital (CAH) is a small Medicare acute care hospital or a health clinic or other facility that was a hospital prior to being converted into a clinic. CAH facilities have to be located more than thirty-five miles from another hospital (15 miles in an area with only secondary roads or in mountainous terrain) unless they were designated as "necessary providers" by the state prior to January 1, 2006. The facilities must provide 24-hour emergency services, have an average length of stay of no more than 96 hours, and be licensed for no more than 25 beds. CAHs are paid based on a percentage of reasonable costs for both inpatient acute care and swing bed services. More information about CAHs is available from CMS (2007a).

Summary

When patients are admitted to healthcare facilities as inpatients, the many services they require are provided by a variety of professionals on the healthcare team. Hospitals in the United States vary according to size, type of ownership, types of services offered, governance structure, and even methodology of reimbursement. It is important to recognize these variances in order to understand the complexity of inpatient treatment.

Chapter 2

Reimbursement Methodologies for Inpatient Services

Over the years, reimbursement for healthcare services has gone through many changes. This chapter focuses on the various types of payment systems used to reimburse hospitals for inpatient services. It also discusses some of the most common payers in the U.S. health system.

Methods of Payment

Typical reimbursement for medical services is paid using several different methods. Some of the most common of those include capitation, fee for service, case rate, per diem, prospective payment system, and fee schedule.

Capitation

Capitation consists of a fixed fee per patient enrolled in the plan. This is considered to be a risk-sharing arrangement because if the patient is extremely sick and requires extensive services, care must be provided without the incentive of additional payment from the patient or the insurance company. Providers must maintain a high quality of care but have to be cost conscious to remain profitable.

Fee for Service

In the fee-for-service payment system, facilities and practitioners are paid for the services provided to the patient without negotiated rates or other forms of cost containment. This form of reimbursement was very common prior to the managed care era of healthcare payment.

Case Rates

A facility that negotiates a contract based on "case rates" is paid a specific amount that is based on the average cost of caring for a patient with a specific disease or service provided.

Per Diem

The term *per diem* means "per day." This form of reimbursement is a fixed rate of payment per day of hospitalization or date of service. It is commonly used in healthcare units such as critical care or skilled nursing units. Usually, a defined list of items is included in the per diem payment rate.

Prospective Payment System

Prospective payment system (PPS) methodology for inpatients involves dividing patients into Medicare Severity Adjusted Diagnosis Related Groups or MS-DRGs. MS-DRGs are used for financial measures but are also a clinical method of dividing patients into groups according to the average cost to care for the patient's condition. These divisions are considered to be both clinically meaningful and statistically valid, meaning that patients in a single group statistically use similar amounts of resources. Although this methodology is used primarily for Medicare inpatient reimbursement (discussed extensively in chapter 3), some other insurance companies have modified the Medicare system for their own payment plans.

Fee Schedules

Physicians and ancillary services such as laboratory and physical therapy services are usually paid based on a fee schedule. A fee schedule is a list of codes and the amount of money the insurance company will pay for each service. If the insurance company pays $3.00 for a urinalysis, for example, that is the total amount the facility will receive regardless of the actual cost of providing the service or the charges submitted.

Reimbursement Arrangements for Healthcare Facilities

The above methods of payment generally illustrate how facilities are paid; the following provides greater detail in the various types of reimbursement arrangements made by insurance carriers. These arrangements typically include fee-based services, managed care, and diagnosis related groups (DRG)-type prospective payment systems.

Fee-Based Services

In the past, most payment was based on charges or actual costs of providing a service. Some insurance companies still reimburse on a fee-based system (fee for service), but this method now is much less common. The fee-based system is also known as retrospective payment because it pays based on the actual charges of providing the services determined after the patient is discharged from the facility.

Insurance plans based on the fee-for-service model are known as indemnity plans. This form of payment was very common prior to managed care, and many experts feel that it caused many of the problems in healthcare reimbursement today. At times, charges were much higher than actual costs to provide services to the patient. Facilities had no incentive to control costs and, in fact, even seemed to be "rewarded" for expensive medical care. Thus, the price of healthcare increased to the point where the healthcare reimbursement industry had to make major changes in order to remain viable. Today, even the existing indemnity plans have adopted some of the concepts commonly used by the managed care community to help control costs, such as preadmission approval and utilization review of services provided. Table 2.1 presents the differences between traditional insurance and managed care.

Table 2.1.   Differences between traditional insurance and managed care

Traditional Insurance	Managed Care
Places restrictions on choice of providers	Encourages or requires use of selected providers
Offers fee-for-service reimbursement of providers	Pays negotiated rates to providers
Functions apart from the healthcare delivery system	Integrates the finance and delivery system
Assumes all financial risk	Shares risk with providers
Offers few financial incentives to control costs	Creates financial incentives for providers and enrollees to control costs
Takes no interest in measuring quality and appropriateness of services	Participates actively in methods to measure quality and monitor appropriateness of care
Has no real budget for cost of services, simply "pay as you go"	Establishes budget for cost of services, prepayment of a fixed premium in many cases

Managed Care Payment Systems

Managed care payment systems, or managed care organizations (MCOs), are capitated payment plans in which all services are provided to the patient for a fixed monthly premium. MCOs include health maintenance organizations (HMOs), preferred provider organizations (PPOs), and point-of-service (POS) plans, which are structured differently but share the following characteristics:

- Rigorous utilization review

- Monitoring and analysis of physicians' practice patterns

- Use of primary care physicians and other caregivers to manage patients

- Steering of patients to high-quality, efficient providers

- Quality improvement programs

- Reimbursement systems that make physicians, hospitals, and other providers financially accountable for the cost and quality of medical services (HIAA 1995)

Health Maintenance Organizations

Typical HMO plans share the "risk" with their physicians. In other words, a percentage of the fixed per patient fee is held back from the physician's payment until the end of the year when the practice can determine how profitable it was. This serves as an incentive plan for the practitioners to exercise greater cost control while maintaining a high quality of care level for the plan's members. Patients may lose some freedom of choice because the facilities and providers are limited to those in the HMO plan, but they usually have lower premiums than with some other forms of insurance coverage and do not have to worry about individual visit copayments or deductibles.

There are typically five types of HMO models:

1.   Group model

2.   Independent provider model

3. Network model

4. Staff model

5. Direct Contact Model (Monsees 2008)

Each of these models is discussed in the following subsections.

Group Model

Under the group model, the HMO contracts with a group of physicians and hospitals to provide services to its patients at a specified rate. Physicians are not employees of the HMO and are free to see patients outside the HMO contract. Instead of being paid for each office visit or service, the physician is paid on a fixed (capitated) fee per patient enrolled in the program.

Independent Provider Model

Independent provider models exist with several different meanings for the acronym IPA: individual practice association, independent physician association, independent practice association, and independent provider association. This form of HMO consists of a group of physicians who form together as a legal corporation (the IPA) to provide care for the HMO patients. The IPA then contracts with individual physicians to provide services for the patients in their existing practice. Payment for these services may be arranged on a fee-for-service or a per capita basis. The IPA form of HMO is typically less costly to set up because it uses physicians who already have established practice sites.

An IPA where physicians and hospital(s) join together to provide contracted services is known as a physician–hospital organization (PHO). In a PHO, both the hospital and the physician practices share in the risk associated with prepayment of services.

Network Model

The network model HMO works with contracts between the HMO and multiple hospitals and physician groups to provide a "network" of services for its members. These mixed-type HMOs contract with multiple groups or IPAs to provide a variety of benefits and allow for greater numbers of affiliated physicians and/or hospitals. Patients enjoy more flexibility and greater freedom to choose providers while staying within their HMO network.

Staff Model

In the staff model HMO, physicians and other healthcare providers are paid employees of the HMO group, which allows for greater cost control over services provided. They typically share office space, medical records, and other services that are provided only to members of the HMO. Most of the physicians and other practitioners are paid on a salary basis, but in some HMOs, they are paid based on established incentive plans.

Direct Contact Model

In a direct contact model, physicians contract with the HMO but may treat patients in their own offices or clinics. Patients choose a "gatekeeper" or primary care physician (PCP). If the patient needs a specialist, the primary care physician refers him or her to a specialist who is also contracted and approved by the HMO.

In 1973, a federal law was enacted called the HMO Act. This law established standard qualifications for HMOs, including type of structure, financial requirements, marketing specifications, and delivery of healthcare. To achieve the status of being federally qualified, HMOs must meet the requirements set forth in the act. The HMO Act was supposed to provide for organizational structure and sound financial backing to ensure the protection of patients. In addition, it was set up to encourage the establishment of more HMO plans. Although HMOs are very common in some parts of the country, they did not become the practice standard that was anticipated.

The story of Kaiser Permanente provides a real-world look at how the group model HMO developed. During the Great Depression, physician Dr. Sidney Garfield had a small practice caring for workers building a huge aqueduct in the middle of the Mojave Desert. A strong believer in preventive care, Dr. Garfield borrowed money to build a small hospital for his patients. An insurance salesman, Harold Hatch, saw that by providing a fixed fee to the hospital per worker on an upfront basis, everyone would benefit. Workers signed up for this plan at the rate of five cents per day, thus beginning a new concept of prepayment for medical services. Henry Kaiser heard about this project and hired Dr. Garfield to provide care for his 6,500 workers building the Grand Coulee Dam in Washington State. The project proved so successful that, in 1945, the Permanente Health Plan was opened to the public with huge support from labor unions. Today, Kaiser Permanente is the largest nonprofit health plan in the U.S., with more than eight million members in ten different states. The company owns more than 30 hospitals and more than 400 medical practices and has approximately 13,000 physicians in its network, providing a wide range of benefit choices for its members (Kaiser Permanente n.d.).

Preferred Provider Organizations

The PPO is a plan that is similar to the group HMO model. PPOs are agreements among groups consisting of hospitals, physicians, and other providers who contract with payers to provide healthcare services at a discounted rate for their members. They are not as strict as traditional HMOs in that, for a higher fee, they allow patients to go outside their network of physicians to receive medical care and they do not have as many risk-sharing incentive plans governing pay for their physicians. Most PPOs include the following elements in their services:

- Limitations exist on the number of providers, and providers must meet specific criteria to become affiliated with the PPO, such as quality of care, fellowship or other credential requirements, and scope of practice.

- Network physicians agree to accept a specific reimbursement level for services provided.

- Utilization review procedures are established and must be followed by the network physicians (HIAA 1995).

Point-of-Service Plans

Some HMOs have expanded their offerings to include more choices for their members, such as the ability to go out of network under certain circumstances. Such plans, known as point-of-service (POS) plans, allow patients to go out of network for a higher copayment rate and/or higher deductible.

Prospective Payment Systems

Laws requiring new payment methodologies have been in place for Medicare systems since the mid-1980s. These systems, called prospective payment systems (PPSs), call for reimbursement based on the average cost to treat patients in a particular category rather than the actual costs incurred in treating the patient. Patients are divided into groups such as MS-DRGs (as discussed above) based on the diagnoses and procedures used to treat their conditions. Medicare is the primary payer that utilizes PPSs, but many other payers reimburse facilities based on a modified method of PPS. (Medicare's PPS systems for inpatient services are discussed in chapters 3 and 4.)

Other Common Methods of Cost Control

Additional methods are used by most of the different types of insurers to help control costs. Some of the most common are pay for performance, preadmission review, utilization review, case management, and retrospective review of services provided.

Pay for Performance/Value Based Purchasing

Medicare has instituted a "Pay for Performance" (P4P) initiative to encourage:

> . . . improved quality of care in all health care settings where Medicare beneficiaries receive their health care services, including physicians' offices and ambulatory care facilities, hospitals, nursing homes, home health care agencies and dialysis facilities (CMS 2007b)

The Centers for Medicare & Medicaid Services (CMS) collaborated with a number of organizations including the National Quality Forum, The Joint Commission, the National Committee for Quality Assurance (NCQA), the Agency for Health Care Research and Quality (AHRQ), and the American Medical Association and their Quality Improvement Organizations (QIO) to develop pay-for-performance initiatives to support quality improvement. For example, hospitals must collect and report data on specific quality measures in order to receive full payment update to their Medicare MS-DRG payments (CMS 2007b).

According to CMS (2007c):

> The Centers for Medicare & Medicaid Services (CMS) has articulated a vision for health care quality—*the right care for every person every time*. To achieve this vision, CMS is committed to care that is safe, effective, timely, patient-centered, efficient, and equitable. Medicare's current payment systems reward quantity, rather than quality of care, and provide neither incentive nor support to improve quality of care. Value-based purchasing (VBP), which links payment more directly to the quality of care provided, is a strategy that can help to transform the current payment system by rewarding providers for delivering high quality, efficient clinical care. Through a number of public reporting programs, demonstration projects, pilot programs, and voluntary efforts, CMS has launched VBP initiatives in hospitals, physician offices, nursing homes, home health services, and dialysis facilities.

Preadmission Review

Preadmission review is the practice of reviewing the circumstances for admission before the patient enters the hospital to assess medical necessity and to ensure coverage. Prior to either elective or nonemergent admissions to the hospital, the facility is required to contact the insurance provider to receive verification of coverage. At this time, the insurance provider may review established criteria to see if the patient's condition requires a hospital admission or if another level of service would be more appropriate for the patient's care. During this process, the insurer may specify the number of days that will be covered under the patient's policy. If the patient requires an extended stay, the hospital and/or physician must obtain approval for the additional coverage.

Utilization Review

Utilization review (UR) is another very popular method of cost control for insurance companies as well as an internal hospital control mechanism. UR is performed by either a nursing professional or a health information management (HIM) professional who is skilled in evaluating health record documentation. The UR professional monitors for documentation completeness in the chart and notifies the physician if the patient's condition or treatment is not supported. Because this process is completed while the patient is still an inpatient, any problems can be addressed during the stay. Typically, the reviewer is checking for appropriate level of care, medical necessity of procedures performed, and need for hospitalization.

Case Management

Case managers may perform services similar to those of the utilization reviewer, but they typically manage the care of more problematic patient cases, such as patients recovering from heart surgery. Case managers frequently use critical paths or care plans established by their medical staff to ensure that the patient's recovery is maximized in order to make the best use of the inpatient hospitalization time frame. They also work with social services to arrange for discharge planning, including skilled nursing and home care as needed by the patient.

Retrospective Review

Many carriers review the patient's health record after he or she is discharged from the hospital. This is called a retrospective review. Commonly, the reviewer uses established criteria to see if the patient met certain standards of care for both severity of illness and intensity of service. If the carrier determines that the patient's record does not reflect the need for the acute admission, it may request a refund for payment for the services.

Common Payers

Many different entities pay for healthcare in the United States, and this section discusses some of the most common payers. These include Medicare, Medicaid, military/veterans, and commercial carriers.

Medicare

Medicare was initially designed in the 1960s to provide catastrophic coverage for older Americans who had worked and paid into the Social Security system. It was not designed to be the full-coverage insurance plan that it has evolved into today. It has changed over the years to include other individuals such as those with disabilities and those with end-stage renal disease. Moreover, it has been modified by Congress to include more preventive care such as cancer screening. The government agency that oversees the Medicare program is the Centers for Medicare and Medicaid Services (CMS). The Medicare Prescription Drug, Improvement, and Modernization Act (MMA) of 2003 was one of the latest significant changes in Medicare.

The Medicare Prospective Payment System

As recently as the 1980s, the following scenario was not uncommon: A family member (for example, Grandma) was bedridden and living at home. When the family wanted to go on vacation, they dropped Grandma off at the hospital on the way out of town for what was commonly referred to as respite care. Because of the lack of regulations surrounding Medicare payment, this type of scenario occurred even when there was no acute medical condition that would necessitate Grandma being treated in an acute care facility.

When Medicare was first developed, it paid claims to hospitals based on the fee-for-service reimbursement plan. The patient was admitted to the hospital where tests and other procedures were performed based on physician orders. After the patient went home, the hospital submitted a bill to Medicare, which paid based on a percentage of the total charges.

This type of indemnity plan actually served to reward physicians and hospitals for overutilization of services. Basically, when the doctor ordered a test, it was performed and Medicare paid the bill with little or no review of the appropriateness or need for the services rendered. After a few years of this type of payment system, it became clear that the Medicare system was in jeopardy of running out of funding. The government soon realized that the Medicare program would not survive unless changes were made to the system. Consequently, the government started searching for ways to maintain better control over the system. It was at this time that the concept of a PPS was first discussed.

Today, the family in the scenario above would have multiple options for taking care of Grandma, but if she did not meet criteria that justified an acute care admission, she would not be placed in the hospital for respite care. Today, not just Medicare, but most insurance companies require a thorough preadmission assessment to allow patients to be cared for in the setting most appropriate for their conditions.

Characteristics of a Prospective Payment System

Several key components characterize a system based on prospectively set prices, including the following:

- Payment rates are established in advance and fixed for the fiscal period to which they apply.
- Payment rates are not automatically determined by the hospital's past or current actual cost.
- Rates represent full payment for services provided.
- The hospital retains the profit or suffers the loss resulting from the difference between the rate of payment and the hospital's cost of caring for the patient.

Typically, the fiscal period mentioned above refers to the government's fiscal year (FY), which runs from October 1 to September 30. However, some of the newer payment systems are set up on other FYs, such as July 1 through June 30. At times, because of errors or changes in technology, some modifications are made to the payment systems quarterly or as needed throughout the year.

Under a PPS reimbursement system, there is a strong incentive for the facility to provide high-quality care at the lowest possible cost. There has been an increase in the use of utilization review professionals and case managers to review the charts during the hospital encounter to ensure that the patient's care is being managed effectively. Prospective payment monitoring also has helped facilities to ensure that services provided are necessary for the patient at the acute level of care.

Because of many legislative changes in the Medicare system over the past twenty years, most types of Medicare services now are paid for under some sort of prospective payment methodology. PPSs exist today in all the following settings:

- Inpatient acute care hospitals

- Outpatient hospitals

- Physician offices

- Skilled nursing facilities

- Long-term care hospitals

- Home healthcare settings

- Inpatient rehabilitation facilities

- Inpatient psychiatric facilities

Chapter 4 contains detailed discussions of the different PPSs and payment groups currently in effect.

Medicare Programs

Medicare enrollees are known as beneficiaries. Beneficiaries are typically patients older than age 65, but others who may qualify for Medicare benefits, such as the disabled, are specified in the Social Security Act. Medicare is divided into four main parts (Medicare Parts A through D), each covering different services.

Medicare contracts with local insurance companies to provide services for Medicare beneficiaries in the area. These contractors manage the Medicare program for a specific geographic area of the country and must follow national coverage determinations (NCDs) as set forth by Medicare. They also can establish local policies for items not addressed in the federal guidelines. The contractors may issue two types of documents:

- Local Coverage Determinations (LCDs) document a decision by the contractor (carrier or fiscal intermediary) whether to cover a particular service.

- Local Medical Review Policies (LMRPs) are administrative and educational tools to assist providers, physicians, and suppliers in submitting correct claims for payment.

LMRPs typically include more information than LCDs on diagnoses that document medical necessity. Most carriers are phasing out the LMRPs and are including more specific information in their LCD policies. Corporate hospitals and groups that have facilities in multiple regions of the U.S. may all be assigned to the same contractor.

Medicare Administrative Contractors

In 2011, Medicare plans to simplify payment structure by discontinuing "carrier" and "fiscal intermediary" designations and designating Regional Medicare Administrative Contractors (MACs). According to the Medicare Benefit Policy Manual:

> Through implementation of Medicare Contracting Reform, CMS will integrate the administration of Medicare Parts A and B for the fee-for-service benefit to new entities called Medicare

Administrative Contractors (MACs). This operational integration will centralize information once held separately, creating a platform for advances in the delivery of comprehensive care to Medicare beneficiaries (CMS 2007a).

Medicare Part A

Medicare Part A pays for inpatient hospitalization and some skilled aftercare services, such as nursing home, home health, and hospice care for covered beneficiaries. The contractor that pays the bills and sets policies for Medicare Part A claims is known as a fiscal intermediary (FI). Medicare patients have maximum benefit periods of 60 full days plus 30 days of coinsurance coverage. This is renewable after the patient has not been in a hospital or skilled nursing facility for 60 days. Patients also have a lifetime reserve benefit of 60 additional days. Moreover, Medicare patients have a lifetime maximum of 190 inpatient psychiatric days of coverage.

Medicare Part B

Medicare Part B is designed to pay for physician-related services, some outpatient hospital services, durable medical equipment (DME), and supplies. Medicare beneficiaries must pay an additional monthly premium for this coverage. Certain services normally covered under Part A can be paid under Part B claims when patients have exhausted their Part A benefits. The contractor for Part B claims is known as a Medicare carrier. Most physician practices in the state of Tennessee, for instance, are under the carrier jurisdiction of CIGNA Government Services, the Part B Medicare carrier for Tennessee, North Carolina, and Idaho.

DME such as wheelchairs, crutches, and other supplies are covered under the jurisdiction of a durable medical equipment regional carrier (DMERC). There are currently four regional carriers for DME, located in Chicago, Philadelphia, Dallas, and Denver. The DMERCs may have a different set of rules and regulations than the Medicare carrier in the area. When a hospital provides DME services, it must be certified as a medical equipment provider and must follow special billing rules and regulations as set forth by Medicare and maintained by the regional DMERC.

Medicare Part C

Medicare Part C, or Medicare Advantage (MA), is a PPO-type of coverage for Medicare beneficiaries that offers options such as regional PPOs and specialized health plans for certain diagnoses. Medicare uses a statistical model to review the costs incurred for the enrollees to determine predictions for future years' healthcare expenses. This model is known as the principal inpatient diagnostic cost group (PIP-DCG) algorithm, a model designed to calculate each beneficiary's relative risk in terms of overall Medicare expenditures.

Medicare Part D

Medicare Part D represents the Medicare Prescription Drug Plan, which provides assistance to Medicare beneficiaries who incur substantial drug expenses. The plan is voluntary and administered by various contractors. The beneficiary is responsible for an annual deductible and copayments, and Medicare reimburses a percentage of drug costs above established thresholds. During the first years of the plan, patients who had a lower income were eligible for prescription drug benefits, but eventually all Medicare patients who are eligible for Medicare Part A or have Part B coverage also will be eligible for the Medicare prescription drug benefits. Beginning in 2006, beneficiaries have had the following two options for receiving these benefits:

- Patients who chose to remain in the traditional Medicare coverage plans will have the option of joining a prescription drug plan (PDP) to obtain drug benefits for an additional charge.

- Patients can switch over to the MA plan and obtain hospital, physician, and prescription drug benefits from one company. The plan that includes medication coverage is known as Medicare Advantage-Prescription Drug (MA-PD).

Medicaid

Medicaid was established in 1965 by Public Law 89-97 (Title XIX of the Social Security Act) as a jointly funded program between the state and federal governments. The program was set up to care for low-income or indigent patients. However, although it is federally funded, the program is run primarily by the individual states. Eligibility, services provided, and payment rates vary from state to state, but the programs must meet general national guidelines for services. The CMS Medicaid Eligibility Summary defines the following categories of patients as eligible for Medicaid:

- Individuals who meet the requirements for the Aid to Families with Dependent Children (AFDC) program that were in effect in their state on July 16, 1996

- Children younger than age six whose family income is at or below 133 percent of the federal poverty level (FPL)

- Pregnant women whose family income is below 133 percent of the FPL (Services to these women are limited to those related to pregnancy, complications of pregnancy, delivery, and postpartum care.)

- Supplemental Security Income (SSI) recipients in most states (Some states use more restrictive Medicaid eligibility requirements that predate SSI.)

- Recipients of adoption or foster care assistance under Title IV of the Social Security Act

- Special protected groups (typically individuals who lose their cash assistance due to earnings from work or from increased Social Security benefits, but who may keep Medicaid for a period of time)

- All children born after September 30, 1983, who are younger than age 19, in families with incomes at or below the FPL

- Certain Medicare beneficiaries, such as those with low income

Some states have received permission from the federal government to make modifications to the basic Medicaid plans to include uninsurable individuals, the medically needy, and children.

Military Programs

TRICARE (formerly known as the Civilian Health and Medical Program of the Uniformed Services [CHAMPUS]) provides medical coverage for active-duty and retired service members. This coverage applies to members of the seven uniformed services (Army, Air Force, Navy, Marine Corps, Coast Guard, Public Health Service, and the National Oceanic and Atmospheric Administration) and their dependents, as well as individuals whose spouses were killed in action.

TRICARE pays for coverage in facilities other than military hospitals and offers several options, including an HMO-type of coverage system and a fee-based payment system. The

HMO/managed care option is known as TRICARE Prime. TRICARE Extra is a PPO option, and TRICARE Standard is a fee-for-service plan. At this time, active-duty members are only eligible for the TRICARE Prime option. TRICARE Plus is a variation of the plan used to cover services in military healthcare facilities when available.

For beneficiaries who are Medicare eligible (age 65 and older), there is also a TRICARE for Life plan option. This plan works as a secondary insurance for those who have Medicare Part B. It picks up expenses such as coinsurance and deductible costs after Medicare pays its portion of the bill.

TRICARE for Life uses a DRG-modified system to reimburse facilities for inpatient care. This benefit is available only when the patient is in the hospital for more days than are allowable under the Medicare system. For days 151 and later of a Medicare stay, TRICARE reimburses the hospital the DRG amount minus the patient's additional copayment rate, which is approximately 25 percent of the charges if the hospital is in network. Table 2.2 shows an example of DRG groupings and weights used to determine payment.

Table 2.2.   CHAMPUS weight and threshold summary for FY 2008

DRG Number	Description	CHAMPUS Weight	Arithmetic Mean Length of Stay	Geometric Mean Length of Stay	Short Stay Threshold
1	CRANIOTOMY AGE >17 W CC	3.6780	7.7	5.4	1
2	CRANIOTOMY AGE >17 W/O CC	2.4731	3.9	3	1
3	CRANIOTOMY AGE 0–17	2.1567	5.8	3.3	1
4	NO LONGER VALID	–	–	–	–
5	NO LONGER VALID	–	–	–	–
6	CARPAL TUNNEL RELEASE	0.8780*	3.1	2.1	1
7	PERIPH & CRANIAL NERVE & OTHER NERV SYST PROC W CC	2.2612	6.5	3.8	1
8	PERIPH & CRANIAL NERVE & OTHER NERV SYST PROC W/O CC	1.6195	2.6	1.9	1
9	SPINAL DISORDERS & INJURIES	1.4173	6.4	3.6	1
10	NERVOUS SYSTEM NEOPLASMS W CC	1.3704	5.6	4	1
11	NERVOUS SYSTEM NEOPLASMS W/O CC	0.8756	3.9	2.5	1
12	DEGENERATIVE NERVOUS SYSTEM DISORDERS	1.0711	5.6	3.8	1
13	MULTIPLE SCLEROSIS & CEREBELLAR ATAXIA	0.9206	4.4	3.6	1
14	INTRACRANIAL HEMORRHAGE OR CEREBRAL INFARCTION	1.3807	4.9	3.6	1
15	NONSPECIFIC CVA & PRECEREBRAL OCCLUSION W/O INFARCT	1.0239	3	2.3	1
16	NONSPECIFIC CEREBROVASCULAR DISORDERS W CC	1.3768	4.9	3.6	1
17	NONSPECIFIC CEREBROVASCULAR DISORDERS W/O CC	0.7734	2.6	2.1	1
18	CRANIAL & PERIPHERAL NERVE DISORDERS W CC	1.0484	5	3.8	1
19	CRANIAL & PERIPHERAL NERVE DISORDERS W/O CC	0.7513	2.8	2.2	1

The healthcare plan for veterans is the Civilian Health and Medical Program of the Department of Veterans Affairs (CHAMPVA). This plan consists of comprehensive coverage where both the veteran and the VA pay a portion of covered healthcare expenses.

According to the Department of Veterans Affairs,

CHAMPVA is a health care benefits program for the spouse or widow(er) and for the children of a veteran who:

1. Is rated permanently and totally disabled due to a service-connected disability by a VA regional office
2. Was rated permanently and totally disabled due to a service-connected condition at the time of death
3. Died of a service-connected disability
4. Died on active duty; and the dependents are not otherwise eligible for DoD TRICARE benefits (VA 2007).

In addition, a Medicare secondary plan called CHAMPVA for Life is available for those covered beneficiaries who are age 65 and older.

Commercial and Nonprofit Group Medical Insurance Plans

Group medical insurance plans are usually purchased through or by an employer. Some patients who cannot qualify for individual insurance plans because of preexisting conditions can obtain insurance through employer-sponsored group plans.

Self-employed individuals or those who work in a group that does not provide group insurance may be eligible to obtain individual medical insurance. These types of policies may cost more than group plans and may contain strict regulations, such as a preexisting clause. Patients who have medical conditions deemed to have existed at the time of coverage do not receive benefits related to those preexisting conditions for a specified time frame after coverage begins.

Insurance companies provide various types of healthcare coverage options and benefits for their customers. For example, a review of a major Blue Cross and Blue Shield program shows that it offers the following options:

- *Major medical:* This option is usually a fee-for-service plan as discussed above. Although patients enjoy greater flexibility in the types of services and the number of providers to choose from, major medical plans tend to be the most expensive for the patient, with higher deductibles and out-of-pocket expenses.

- *Preferred payment plan:* The preferred payment plan is a PPO-type system in which members have a more limited number of providers to select from based on negotiated contracts with the facilities and physician practices. They may include a POS option, allowing the beneficiary to go out of network for a reduced percentage of reimbursement.

- *Hospital reimbursement program:* The hospital reimbursement program is used for reimbursement for hospital inpatient stays. The hospital agrees to accept a DRG-type payment methodology in which the payment received is considered as payment in full. The beneficiary will incur no costs other than the deductible and copayment amounts. This plan is similar to the DRG system utilized in the Medicare inpatient PPS.

- *COBRA and HIPAA benefits:* Patients who have group insurance and leave their jobs or are laid off are usually eligible to keep their insurance coverage up to 18 months after their employment ends but are required to pay the premiums in order to keep the coverage intact. These benefits are provided by federal law under the Consolidated Omnibus Budget Reconciliation Act of 1986 (COBRA). Continuation of coverage is only effective under specific circumstances, such as loss of a job or life events such as death or divorce. Typically, COBRA is in effect for employers who offer group healthcare and have twenty or more employees.

The Health Insurance Portability and Accountability Act of 1996 (HIPAA) allows for healthcare coverage protection for those who move or change jobs, although the premiums for these policies are often very expensive. HIPAA also prohibits group plans from either denying coverage or charging extra due to current or past medical history. There is usually a limited or no preexisting clause in the HIPAA insurance plan. Patients have to show that they have a minimum of 18 months of credible coverage of previous insurance without significant break (no more than 63 days in a row without insurance) to be eligible for HIPAA insurance.

Summary

Various methods of payment are used to reimburse facilities that provide services to inpatients. Although Medicare's DRG system is probably the most widely studied, other payment methodologies such as HMOs are very prevalent in many sections of the country. The wide variety of payment methodologies can be a source of confusion for hospital coders, billers, and other finance personnel, so it is very important to understand these systems and their impact on the financial well-being of the healthcare facility.

Chapter 3

Structure and Organization of the Medicare Inpatient Acute Care Prospective Payment System

The Social Security Act, as amended in 1982 by the Tax Equity and Fiscal Responsibility Act (TEFRA), mandated the use of a prospective payment system (PPS) for inpatient hospital services provided under Part A of Medicare. In the 1970s, a research team at Yale University looked into classifying patients into categories based on the diagnoses that caused them to be admitted to the hospital in order to determine why patients with similar cases differed in their usage of resources. Patients were divided into various categories that were medically meaningful in that all patients in the same category would be expected to respond in a clinically similar manner. The data were averaged statistically to show that patients placed in these categories consumed about equal amounts of the hospital's facilities and resources. The categories became known as diagnosis- (or diagnostic-) related groups (DRGs). In fiscal year (FY) 2008 these were revised into Medicare Severity Adjusted DRGs or MS-DRGs. This chapter discusses DRGs, their evolution to MS-DRGs and their role in the development of the PPS inpatient system.

Diagnosis-Related Groups

DRGs are derived from all the diagnoses and procedures listed in the ICD-9-CM classification system. DRGs are simply numbers signifying into which category the patient best fits. Grouping patients into categories that consume similar amounts of resources reveals typical and atypical patterns of utilization. The researchers who developed the DRG system were trying to define expected lengths of patient stays so that utilization review (UR) activities could be focused on atypical patients. Their design was not established with the intent to use it as the basis for a payment system. However, when the government learned of the study, it became interested and funded a project in New Jersey to see if this type of system would work as a reimbursement system.

Simply defined, a DRG is a group of clinically coherent conditions with a similar pattern of resource intensity determined by the principal diagnosis, significant additional diagnoses (and their present-on-admission status), and procedures as reported on the Uniform Bill-04 (UB-04) (Kennedy 2008).

Development of the Inpatient PPS System

Section 1886(d) of the Social Security Act (the Act) sets forth a system of payment for the operating costs of acute care hospital inpatient stays under Medicare Part A (Hospital Insurance) based on prospectively set rates. Section 1886(g) of the Act requires the Secretary to pay for the capital-related costs of hospital inpatient stays under a prospective payment system (PPS). Under these PPSs, Medicare payment for hospital inpatient operating and capital-related costs is made at predetermined, specific rates for each hospital discharge" (CMS2007d, 47135). Hospitals subject to the prospective payment system are paid a specific amount for each discharge based on the case's classification into a DRG. Every hospital discharge case fits into a DRG category. A hierarchy has been established to ensure that each case fits only into one category group.

The DRGs provide classification for the complete range of diagnoses represented in the ICD-9-CM codebook.

Because assignment of a case to a particular DRG determines the amount that will be paid for the case, it is important that the assignment be done in a systematic and uniform manner. According to the Centers for Medicare and Medicaid Services (CMS), the following core elements are included in a PPS-type system (CMS 2008a):

- The base payment amount

- A "wage index," which reflects that labor costs vary in different areas of the country

- The standardized weights that are established to compare the average resources needed to care for patients in each DRG

- Additional payments for those hospitals with treatment patterns that fall into specific categories, such as:

    —A large share of low-income or indigent patients

    —Teaching hospitals to reflect the higher cost of providing medical education

    —Additional payment for very high-cost patients, known as outliers

Grouper Software

To meet this objective, CMS established the grouper program, which is an automated classification system that uses the prescribed information to assign discharges to their proper DRGs. The fiscal intermediary (FI)/Medicare Administrative Contractor (MAC), which is the organization contracting with Medicare to process hospital inpatient claims for CMS, assigns the proper DRG using the grouper program. Most hospitals assign DRGs for all cases to facilitate quality management activities and estimate revenue, but it is the DRG assigned by the FI/MACs grouper that determines final reimbursement.

Coding instructions for the PPS indicate that the hospital will submit a bill for a particular case using classifications and terminology consistent with ICD-9-CM and the Uniform Hospital Data Discharge Set (UHDDS) prescribed by the National Committee on Vital and Health Statistics (NCVHS).

According to CMS, the updated MS-DRGs and Grouper software, used by both the inpatient prospective payment system (IPPS) and the LTCH-MS-DRG system are based on updated ICD-9-CM codes in a manner consistent with current usage and the Health Insurance Portability and Accountability Act of 1996 (HIPAA) regulations. Historically, these codes have been published annually in the IPPS proposed rule and final rule but are also available in the *Coding*

Clinic for ICD-9-CM published by the American Hospital Association. This brief offers official coding advice for the coder about which ICD-9-CM instructions and UHDDS sequencing guidelines apply when coding for the PPS.

DRG Variables

A patient is assigned to only one DRG group per admission. Because many patients have multiple diagnoses and procedures, a classification hierarchy had to be incorporated into the system. Patients originally were assigned to a DRG based on the following variables:

- Principal diagnosis, if no qualifying surgery is performed

- Secondary diagnoses

- Principal or significant procedure

- Age

- Sex

- Patient status (discharge disposition)

Principal Diagnosis

The principal diagnosis is defined in the UHDDS as "that condition established after study to be chiefly responsible for occasioning the admission of the patient to the hospital for care" (HHS 1985). This helps to establish a standard definition when comparing data from different facilities but causes much confusion in coding. For example, if a patient is admitted with chest pain, and after testing it is determined that the patient is suffering from an acute myocardial infarction (AMI), the AMI qualifies as the principal diagnosis. However, if the patient is admitted for treatment of benign prostate hypertrophy and then after admission has a massive heart attack, even though the focus of the admission has changed, the principal diagnosis is the prostate condition with the heart attack meeting the definition for additional diagnosis reporting.

It can be confusing for the coder to distinguish between the "principal" diagnosis and the most "significant additional diagnosis." UHDDS defines additional diagnoses as "all conditions that coexist at the time of admission, that develop subsequently, or that affect the treatment received and/or the length of stay" (HHS 1985).

Secondary Diagnoses

According to the UHDDS, secondary diagnoses include all conditions that "coexist at the time of admission, or develop subsequently, which affect the treatment received and/or the length of stay. Diagnoses that refer to an earlier episode that have no bearing on the current hospital or nursing home stay are to be excluded. Conditions should be coded that affect patient care in terms of requiring clinical evaluation; therapeutic treatment; diagnostic procedures; extended length of hospital or nursing home stay; or increased nursing care and/or monitoring" (HHS 1985). Secondary diagnoses may help to determine the grouping if they qualify as a complication or comorbidity (CC). Statistically, a CC is a "condition, which because of its presence with a specific principal diagnosis, would cause an increase in the length of stay by at least one day in at least 75 percent of the patients" (CMS 2007d, 47240). Complications are those conditions that arise after admission. If a patient is admitted with pneumonia and then has a stroke on the second day of hospitalization, the stroke would be considered a complication according to the UHDDS definition. This definition may not be the same as a complication due to, or caused by, a surgical or medical procedure. Comorbidities are conditions that are present on admission, such as a systemic disease like Type II diabetes or essential hypertension, or concomitant acute illnesses or injuries. These illnesses may cause a patient to recover at a slower rate than a patient without any additional problems. In the case of paired DRGs, a single CC (complication or comorbid condition) can cause the patient's case to be grouped into the higher-weighted MS-DRG.

For FY 2008, Medicare made major revisions to the CC list and then divided these into CC and MCC (major CC) lists. The definition of CC had not changed since it was first established at the onset of the DRG system. However, there have been many changes impacting the patients that have been admitted to the hospital. In 1983, the average length of stay for Medicare patients was 9.8 days, and by 2005 it had dropped to 5.7 days. Changes in practice patterns and an increase in postacute care services as well as a shift to performing more services in the outpatient area has meant that patients who are admitted to the hospital are much sicker than they were in the past. Subsequently, by 2005, approximately 80 percent of Medicare patients admitted to U.S. hospitals had a secondary condition that counted as a CC (CMS 2007d, 47153). In FY 2007 there were 115 MS-DRGs split based on the presence or absence of CC, and Medicare decided it was time to reevaluate the types of diagnoses that counted as CCs.

Chronic Illnesses

The presence of a chronic illness does not automatically mean that the patient will need to stay in the hospital longer. Some chronic illnesses do not impact length of stay unless they are associated with an acute exacerbation or significant deterioration in the underlying chronic condition. Medicare reviewed chronic illnesses and removed several of them from the CC list, including congestive heart failure (CHF) and chronic obstructive pulmonary disease (COPD). Another example of this is Mitral Valve Disease. Up through FY 2007, codes 396.0-396.9 were included on the CC list. Unless these diagnoses are combined with other diagnoses showing acute deterioration such as acute heart failure, acute pulmonary edema, or respiratory failure, they will not necessarily impact the patient's length of stay or resources necessary to care for the patient. Therefore, these codes are not on the revised CC list for FY 2008.

Advanced Chronic Illnesses

For those conditions that are divided into stages of illnesses, only those stages or levels of severity that impact length of stay and/or resources used are counted as CCs. For example, a patient with chronic kidney disease is staged according to the level of glomerular filtration rate (GFR). Stages I-III are not counted as CCs, but stages IV, V (kidney failure) or end-stage renal disease (ESRD) are counted as CCs. If a patient is diagnosed with morbid obesity, it will only count as a CC if paired with a body mass index (BMI) of greater than 35.

Codes Where Stage Not Specified

For chronic conditions where the stage is not specified, the conditions were evaluated based on the consistency and intensity of the debility or decompensation associated with the illness. Quadriplegia, for example, is always considered significant, so it counts as a CC when coded as a secondary diagnosis.

Acute Diagnosis Codes

Acute conditions that always impact length of stay (LOS) and/or amount of resources used remained on the CC list. Examples include:

- Acute myocardial infarction (AMI) (not CC if already impacts MS-DRG assignment)
- Cerebrovascular accident (CVA)
- Acute respiratory failure
- Pneumonia
- Septicemia

Other acute conditions were included based on their impact on hospital resource usage. If they were found to be comparable to these listed diagnoses, then they were left on the CC list, but if not, they were removed. For example, acute endocarditis remained on the CC list, but urinary tract infection (UTI) was removed.

Revised CC List

In summary, secondary conditions only count as CCs if they have been found to have consistently greater impact on hospital resources and include the following:

- Significant acute diseases
- Acute exacerbation of significant chronic illnesses
- Advanced or end stage chronic illnesses
- Chronic diseases associated with extensive debility

For FY 2008, this reduced the number of secondary codes that count as CCs from 3,326 to 2,583 codes and should reduce the number of inpatients with CCs to approximately 40.34 percent.

CC Exclusion List

Medicare also has developed a listing of CC exclusions. Some secondary diagnoses may act as CCs with certain diagnoses, but not with others. For example, urinary retention is on the standard CC list, but if present with benign prostatic hyperplasia (BPH), it is excluded as a CC because it is considered to be an integral part of the clinical presentation of BPH. As such, it does not cause an increase in the amount of resources needed to care for the patient. Medicare places codes on the CC exclusion list based on one of these five reasons (CMS 2007d, 47240):

1. Chronic and acute manifestations of the same condition should not be considered CCs for one another.

2. Specific and nonspecific (that is, not otherwise specified [NOS]) diagnosis codes for the same condition should not be considered CCs for one another.

3. Codes for the same condition that cannot coexist, such as partial/total, unilateral/bilateral, obstructed/unobstructed, and benign/malignant, should not be considered CCs for one another.

4. Codes for the same condition in anatomically proximal sites should not be considered CCs for one another.

5. Closely related conditions should not be considered CCs for one another.

Other Factors Influencing DRG Assignment

In some cases in the past, other factors such as age, sex, and discharge status have affected DRG assignment. For example, if patients in one age group tended to use more resources than patients in another age group, the DRGs were split according to age. (This was eliminated in FY 2008 with the onset of MS-DRGs). Sex is used primarily to indicate a keystroke error such as a hysterectomy patient classified as a male patient. Discharge status is a factor in the facility obtaining partial DRG payment when the patient is transferred to another facility or when a certain type of discharge status shows a statistical difference in the amount of resources utilized. Medicare's postacute care transfer policy allows for a decrease in payment if postacute care treatment related to the hospital admission occurs following the patient's discharge. This policy is discussed in detail later in this chapter. Figure 3.1 presents a flowchart of the of DRG process.

Major Diagnostic Categories and Surgical Hierarchy

Before patients' admissions are divided into DRGs, they are divided into MDCs, or major diagnostic categories. Each MDC is based on major body systems and contains multiple DRGs.

Figure 3.1. Flowchart of the MS-DRG process

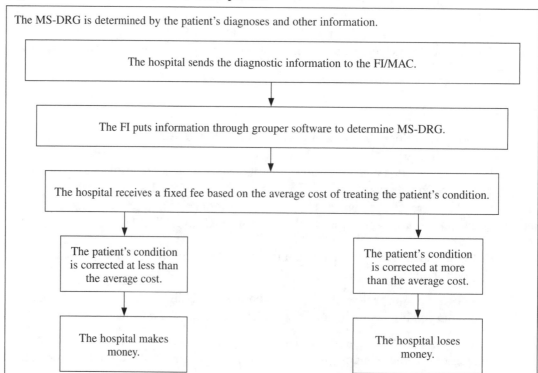

There were originally 23 MDCs and 470 DRGs. These are reviewed and adjusted each year. As of FY 2008, there are 25 major diagnostic categories, one category of diagnoses and procedures associated with all MDCs (including mostly ungroupable diagnoses and procedures) and one pre-MDC, composed only of surgical DRGs related primarily to organ transplants. DRGs within each MDC are separated into medical and surgical divisions. When more than one procedure is performed, the DRG that is highest according to the surgical hierarchy in the MDC is assigned. For example under the MS-DRG system in MDC 5, diseases and disorders of the circulatory system, MS-DRG 242, permanent cardiac pacemaker implant with MCC, takes precedence over MS-DRG 247, percutaneous cardiovascular procedure with drug-eluting stent or AMI without MCC. If a patient has both types of procedures during a single admission, he or she would be grouped into MS-DRG 242 according to the surgical hierarchy.

DRG Relative Weight

Each DRG is assigned a relative weight that represents the average resources required to care for a patient assigned to a specific DRG in relation to the national average of resources used to treat all Medicare cases. When DRG groups were first developed, there needed to be a way to compare the different groups according to the amount of resources utilized. To obtain a starting point for comparison, the average cost of all Medicare patients was established and assigned a relative weight of 1.0000. All patient cases then were divided into DRGs and ranked in order according to the number of resources utilized. As all other DRGs were compared to the average, they were assigned weights appropriate for their average resources used by patients in that group. For example, if one DRG takes twice as many resources as the average, it would be weighted at 2.0000. Conversely, if a group takes half as many resources as average, it would be weighted at 0.5000. Weights for all DRGs are updated every year and published in the *Federal Register,* with the changes becoming effective on October 1 of each year. Relative weights for FY 2008 MS-DRGs range from a high of 23.1117 for MS-DRG 001 (pre-MDC), heart transplant or implant of heart assist system with MCC to a low of 0.1580 for MS-DRG 795 (MDC 15), Normal Newborn.

Adjustment to the Facility Payment Rate

Although the DRG weight is the same for all facilities, hospitals may receive different payment rates based on several factors, including labor costs, disproportionate-share hospitals, medical education, new technology, and other factors.

Labor Costs

The DRG amount is divided into labor- and non-labor-related costs. To account for differences in the labor portion, Medicare established wage areas throughout the different regions of the country. In other words, it costs more to hire staff in some areas of the country than in others, so hospitals are compensated for that additional expense. In Alaska and Hawaii, the rate also is adjusted for the area's cost of living. For example, for FY 2008, the wage indexes for the main areas of Tennessee are as shown in table 3.1.

Occupational Mix Adjustment

Every three years Medicare collects data to determine how occupational mix adjustment impacts wages. According to CMS, "the purpose of the occupational mix adjustment is to control for the effect of hospitals' employment choices on the wage index. For example, hospitals may choose to employ different combinations of registered nurses, licensed practical nurses, nursing aides, and medical assistants for the purpose of providing nursing care to their patients. The varying labor costs associated with these choices reflect hospital management decisions rather than geographic differences in the costs of labor" (CMS 2007d, 47309). Hospitals are required to complete a survey that includes data regarding specific wages, hours, and types of personnel employed in certain job types.

Disproportionate-Share Hospitals

Hospitals that treat a high number of low-income patients may receive an additional amount per case known as their disproportionate-share hospital (DSH) adjustment. An example of DSH adjustments are shown in table 3.2 (CMS 2007d, 47383).

Table 3.1.   FY 2008 wage indexes for Tennessee

Urban Areas	Constituent Counties	Area Wage Index
Jackson, TN	Chester County, TN Madison County, TN	0.8591
Kingsport-Bristol-Bristol, TN-VA (TN Hospitals)	Hawkins County, TN Sullivan County, TN (Bristol City, VA) (Scott County, VA) (Washington County, VA)	0.7917
Knoxville, TN	Anderson County, TN Blount County, TN Knox County, TN Loudon County, TN Union County, TN	0.8012
Memphis, TN-MS-AR	Crittenden County, AR DeSoto County, MS Marshall County, MS Tate County, MS Tunica County, MS Fayette County, TN Shelby County, TN Tipton County, TN	0.9313
Nashville-Davidson-Murfreesboro-Franklin, TN	Cannon County, TN Cheatham County, TN Davidson County, TN Dickson County, TN Hickman County, TN Macon County, TN Robertson County, TN Rutherford County, TN Smith County, TN Sumner County, TN Trousdale County, TN Williamson County, TN Wilson County, TN	0.9618

Source: CMS2007d, 47503–47526.

Table 3.2.   Example of DSH adjustments

Name	Total SSI	Total Medicare	SSI Ratio
Southeast Medical Center	8,278	50,829	0.16286
Marshall Medical Center South	1,931	13,401	0.14409
Eliza Coffee Memorial Hospital	5,042	45,345	0.11119
Mizell Memorial Hospital	1,169	6,635	0.17619
Crenshaw Community Hospital	474	2,469	0.19198
Hartselle Medical Center	463	4,218	0.10977
Marshall Medical Center North	1,712	12,495	0.13701
Medical Center East	1,821	27,619	0.06593
Baptist Dekalb	854	6,668	0.12807

This DSH adjustment was enacted by the Consolidated Omnibus Budget Reconciliation Act (COBRA) to impact discharges beginning in May of 1986. There are two ways for hospitals to qualify to receive this additional amount. The more common way to qualify is through a formula determined in COBRA, which determines a DSH patient percentage by adding the Medicare and Medicaid fractions. According to CMS, the Medicare fraction is (CMS2007d, 47383):

> . . . computed by dividing the number of patient days that are furnished to patients who were entitled to both Medicare Part A and Supplemental Security Income (SSI) benefits by the total number of patient days furnished to patients entitled to benefits under Medicare Part A. The Medicaid fraction is computed by dividing the number of patient days furnished to patients who, for those days, were eligible for Medicaid but were not entitled to benefits under Medicare Part A by the number of total hospital patient days in the same period.

When the DSH patient percentage is greater than 15 percent, the facility is eligible for an additional payment.

Large urban hospitals also can qualify if their total net inpatient care revenue received from state and local governments for indigent care is more than 30 percent. This percentage does not include funds received from either Medicare or Medicaid. According to CMS, hospitals qualifying through this method are known as "Pickle hospitals." Rural hospitals that qualify as rural referral centers or sole community hospitals also may qualify through various formulas established in the law. Rural hospitals with fewer than 500 beds are capped at 12 percent DSH limits but those that qualify as rural referral centers have no cap. A hospital can qualify as a rural referral center if it has more than 275 beds or meets the following two requirements:

1.   A minimum case-mix index that is equal to that of the median case-mix index of urban hospitals in the region or nationally. An example of Medicare median case-mix index is found in table 3.3.

2.   An annual number of discharges of 5,000 or more per year or equal to that of the urban hospitals in the region.

Table 3.3. Medicare-defined median case-mix index (CMI) per region for FY 2008

Region	States	CMI
New England	CT, ME, MA, NH, RI, VT	1.2348
Middle Atlantic	PA, NJ, NY	1.2665
South Atlantic	DE, DC, FL, GA, MD, NC, SC, WV, VA	1.3515
East North Central	IL, IN, MI, OH, WI	1.3393
East South Central	AL, KY, MS, TN	1.2904
West North Central	IA, KS, MN, MO, NE, ND, SD	1.2869
West South Central	AR, OK, LA, TX	1.2869
Mountain	AZ, CO, ID, MT, NV, NM, UT, WY	1.4260
Pacific	AK, CA, HI, OR, WA	1.3772

Source: CMS 2007d, 47368.

Medical Education

Teaching hospitals receive an additional payment for their indirect medical education (IME) costs, which are based on a comparison of hospital residents to number of hospital beds. This provision also was set forth in the COBRA law of 1985. The law takes into account direct-versus-indirect medical education costs. For direct medical education costs, the hospital's per resident amount (PRA) is determined by dividing its allowable costs for education by the number of residents during the time period. The PRA then is multiplied by the number of full-time equivalent (FTE) residents during the reporting period and the hospital's number of inpatient days for Medicare patients.

When PPS hospitals have residents in an approved graduate medical education (GME) program, the hospital obtains additional payment per Medicare discharge for IME costs. The IME adjustment factor compares the number of residents per beds and is multiplied by a rate that is set by Congress. Typically, for each 10 percent increase in resident-to-bed ratio, the facility receives additional funding.

The Balanced Budget Act (BBA), the Balanced Budget Refinement Act (BBRA), and the Benefits Improvement and Protection Act (BIPA) all contained stipulations to allow for modification of the IME multiplier.

New Technology

Another adjustment to the facility's payment rate is based on new technology. At times, Medicare will pay an additional fee for the use of new technology, such as very high-cost medications. According to Medicare (CMS 2007d, 47300):

> A new technology or medical service must demonstrate that it is a substantial clinical improvement over technologies or services otherwise available, and that, absent an add-on payment, it would be inadequately paid under the regular DRG system. For example, a new technology

represents a substantial clinical improvement when it reduces mortality, decreases the number of hospitalizations or physician visits, or reduces recovery time compared to the technologies previously available.

There are specific criteria and rules set up to define what is meant by "new" in the language of the law, which includes the provision of paying for the new technology separately until enough time has passed to allow for sufficient data to be collected on the technology. This is defined as at least two years, but no longer than three years.

For example, endovascular graft repair of the thoracic aorta (GORE TAG), procedure code 39.73 (endovascular implantation of graft in the thoracic aorta) was covered under the new technology payment from FY 2006 through FY 2007. Currently, Medicare pays the DRG payment amount plus 50 percent of the costs of the new technology. Makers of new technology have to formally submit a written proposal to determine if their product will qualify under the new technology regulations.

Other Factors

Other categories of hospitals receive additional payments based on status. Small facilities designated as sole community hospitals (SCHs) and Medicare-dependent rural hospitals (MDHs) are paid based on a formula of DRG rate or on their costs for specific time periods, whichever is higher. When a facility qualifies as an MDH, it is paid 75 percent of the difference between the IPPS rate and the hospital-specific rate when that rate is higher than the IPPS rate for the DRG payment amount. These facilities serve a large Medicare population and are usually located in rural areas. There is no longer a cap on their disproportionate share payment adjustment. SCHs are rural hospitals located at least fifteen miles from other like hospitals, among other requirements. MDH hospitals have fewer than 100 beds and are not classified as SCHs.

Facility Base Rate

Each facility is assigned a base rate that takes into account all these factors. The base rate then is multiplied by the DRG weight to determine the actual payment rate for that facility.

Outliers

When the patient's costs exceed a predetermined cost threshold, the facility may be eligible to receive an additional reimbursement added to the DRG base rate. This patient is known as a cost outlier. If the patient qualifies as an outlier, a determination of additional payment is made, which begins at the cost threshold amount. The hospital's cost-to-charge ratios are used to determine whether a patient's costs are greater than the threshold amount. After the threshold limit (which is $22,650 for FY 2008) is reached, the hospital receives a percentage of costs above this amount.

Hospitals Exempt from Inpatient PPS

These hospitals are paid solely under a reasonable cost-based system. Some facilities are considered to be exempt from the DRG payment system and are paid based on a "reasonable cost-based system" which includes children's hospitals, cancer hospitals, and religious nonmedical healthcare institutions. Other types of facilities that are exempt from the IPPS are now paid based on PPSs specific to their patient populations, such as long-term care hospitals, inpatient psychiatric facilities, and inpatient rehabilitation facilities. The payment methodology for these other systems is discussed in chapter 4.

Transfers

Hospitals must carefully show the patient's discharge status on the billing form because it can have an impact on reimbursement. This is true even of a patient who is transferred from the acute care setting into another unit within the hospital, such as a long-term care or swing bed service.

Because the DRG payment is supposed to pay for all care associated with diagnoses and treatment necessary to care for a patient, when a patient is transferred prior to completion of that care, the DRG payment rate is adjusted to account for the change. For example, when a patient is transferred from one facility that is paid under the IPPS to another facility also paid under the IPPS, the two facilities share the DRG total payment. In the past several years, Medicare has developed a postacute care transfer policy that also adjusts the DRG payment based on incomplete care.

Medicare's postacute care transfer policy distinguishes between discharges and transfers of beneficiaries from inpatient hospitals under the PPS. Consistent with the policy, Medicare pays the full DRG payment to a hospital that discharges an inpatient to home. When a patient is transferred, each transferring hospital is paid a per diem rate for each day of the stay that cannot exceed the full DRG payment that would have been made if the patient had been discharged without being transferred.

In contrast, for specified DRGs, Medicare pays a hospital that transfers an inpatient to certain postacute care settings, such as a skilled nursing facility or home healthcare, a per diem rate for each day of the stay, not to exceed the full DRG payment for a discharge. Twice the per diem amount is paid for the first day of hospitalization. Only certain DRGs are included in the postacute care payment policy.

The purpose of the IPPS postacute care transfer payment policy is to avoid providing an incentive for a hospital to transfer patients to another hospital early in the patients' stay in order to minimize costs while still receiving the full DRG payment. The transfer policy adjusts the payments to approximate the reduced costs of transfer cases.

Beginning with the FY 2006 IPPS, the regulations specified that a DRG is subject to the postacute care transfer policy if the DRG meets the following criteria (CMS 2007d, 47187):

- The DRG had a geometric mean length of stay of at least 3 days;

- The DRG had at least 2,050 postacute care transfer cases; and

- At least 5.5 percent of the cases in the DRG were discharged to postacute care prior to the geometric mean length of stay for the DRG.

- The total number of discharges to postacute care in the DRG must equal or exceed the 55th percentile for all DRGs; and

- The proportion of short-stay discharges to postacute care to total discharges in the DRG exceeds the 55th percentile for all DRGs. A short-stay discharge is a discharge before the geometric mean length of stay for the DRG.

Special Payment Methodology

A transfer is subject to the "special payment methodology" if it is in the same base DRG as any other subcategory that qualifies for special payment methodology, in which the patient is transferred early to a postacute care setting. The payment rate for these types of transfers is 50 percent of the total DRG payment plus the average per diem for the first day of the stay plus 50 percent of the per diem for each subsequent day of the stay not to exceed the full DRG payment.

See table 3.4 for an example of FY 2008 MS-DRGs showing which DRGs fall under the postacute care transfer and special payment methodology policies.

Annual Updates

The IPPS was designed to be modified once each year to allow for updates. The largest update occurs because of the creation, revision, or deletion of ICD-9-CM codes. Also, because the IPPS is based on statistical and medical cohesiveness, there are times when changes need to be made, such as a redistribution of codes to different DRG groupings. These changes are published in the *Federal Register* with an effective date of October 1 of each year. The ICD-9-CM coding system may be updated twice per year (October and April) to allow for the addition of

Table 3.4. **Sample of MS-DRGs, relative weighting factors, and geometric and arithmetic mean LOS**

MS–DRG	FY 2008 Final Rule Post–acute DRG	FY 2008 Final Rule Special Pay DRG	MDC	Type	MS-DRG Title	Weights	Geometric Mean LOS	Arithmetic Mean LOS
001	No	No	PRE	SURG	Heart transplant or implant of heart assist system w MCC.	23.1117	30.8	45.6
002	No	No	PRE	SURG	Heart transplant or implant of heart assist system w/o MCC.	16.2735	16.1	22.8
003	Yes	No	PRE	SURG	ECMO or trach w MV 96+ hrs or PDX exc face, mouth & neck w maj O.R.	18.7707	33.4	40.6
004	Yes	No	PRE	SURG	Trach w MV 96+ hrs or PDX exc face, mouth & neck w/o maj O.R.	11.4219	23.8	29.3
005	No	No	PRE	SURG	Liver transplant w MCC or intestinal transplant.	10.6120	17.6	23.5
006	No	No	PRE	SURG	Liver transplant w/o MCC.	7.2562	9.1	10.5
007	No	No	PRE	SURG	Lung transplant	8.4002	14.6	17.3
008	No	No	PRE	SURG	Simultaneous pancreas/ kidney transplant.	5.1726	10.1	11.8
009	No	No	PRE	SURG	Bone marrow transplant	6.4842	18.1	21.7
010	No	No	PRE	SURG	Pancreas transplant	3.8902	9.2	10.5

Source: CMS 2007d, table 5, 47539.

codes for new technology, but since this rule has been enacted, very few changes have been made midyear. When new codes are added midyear, they are assigned to current DRG groups until the following October, when the DRG groups are updated, as needed.

Severity of Illness

One common criticism of the Medicare DRG system is that the severity of a patient's disease is not always directly reflected in the DRG assignment. In the case of paired DRGs, the presence of a single CC has been shown to significantly add to the resources needed to fully treat the patient. Therefore, patients within one DRG may vary greatly in the number of additional diagnoses they have, meaning that patients in the same DRG could consume quite different quantities of resources. This is supposed to be accounted for in the law of averages, as one patient may use fewer resources for his or her care and one may use more, so theoretically the hospital breaks even. However, research is being conducted on variations of the DRG system to attempt to capture severity of illness data.

Medicare Severity Adjusted DRGs (MS-DRGs)

In order to "more accurately stratify groups of Medicare patients with varying level of severity," Medicare undertook the biggest change to the DRG system since it was established in the 1980s (CMS 2007, 47155). For FY 2008, Medicare revamped the DRG system to incorporate severity of illness into the DRG payment system. While keeping the core elements and modifications made to DRGs over the years, this update should allow for more accurate payment for patients with multiple diagnoses. The first step in revising the DRG system consisted of consolidating DRGs by combining certain DRGs and eliminating all divisions based on age and divisions between "paired" DRGs, such as those divided based on the presence or absence of secondary conditions.

Three Levels of Severity

Medicare then reviewed all diagnoses on the CC list to determine how each impacted length of stay and amount of resources used. The revised CC list was compared with CC lists in the all-patient refined diagnosis-related group (APR-DRG) and all-patient diagnosis-related group (AP-DRG) systems and other severity based revisions of the DRG system. Conditions were divided into three different levels of severity: non-CC, CC, and MCC.

The lowest level was assigned to those diagnoses that do not significantly affect severity of illness and resource usage and are known as "non-CCs." The middle level of severity are known as CCs, and the highest level of severity are deemed MCC or Major CC.

After this secondary diagnosis analysis, the 311 base MS-DRGs were then subdivided into the three CC subcategories with patients assigned to the subgroup with the most extreme CC present. Each base MS-DRG may be subdivided based on the severity of the patient's secondary diagnoses. These three groups are as follows:

1. Patients with no other secondary diagnoses (dx) or with all other secondary dx that are non-CCs

2. Patients with at least one secondary dx that is a CC, but the patient does not have any MCCs.

3. Patients with at least one other secondary dx that is classified as an MCC.

For example, in the category of heart failure, code 428.21 Acute systolic heart failure is considered an MCC, 428.1 left heart failure counts as a CC, and 428.0 Congestive Heart Failure is a non-CC.

Not all base MS-DRGs are subdivided into three different subcategories. CMS established criteria in order to determine the necessity for division of MS-DRGs into CC and MCC subgroups. Those criteria are as follows:

- Reduction in variance of charges of at least 3 percent

- At least 5 percent of patients in the base MS-DRG fall in CC or MCC subgroup

- At least 500 cases are in the CC or MCC subgroup

- At least a 20 percent difference in average charges between subgroups

- $4,000 difference in average charges between subgroups

For FY 2008, there are a total of 745 MS-DRGs. Fifty-three (53) of those are not subdivided into different subgroups and 456 are base groups divided into three subgroups. One hundred and twenty-six (126) MS-DRGs consist of base MS-DRGs divided into two subgroups: MCC and CC in one group and non-CCs in another subgroup, while 86 are made up of two subdivisions: non-CC and CC together and MCC in a separate subgroup. Twenty two consist of mothers and babies in MDC 14 and there are two error MS-DRGs. Spencer and Hyde (2008) provide greater information on the comparisons between the DRG and MS-DRG systems. Some examples are shown in table 3.5.

DRG Modifications

Even though some insurance companies use the DRG methodology for payment purposes, CMS is quick to point out that DRGs are designed to classify the Medicare patient population only. Because of this, revisions have been made over the years to develop systems that groups patients of all types. AP-DRGs group patients of all ages, including the pediatric population, into DRGs based on factors such as birth weight, neonatal age, trauma, and substance abuse.

The APR-DRG methodology was designed by 3M Healthcare and uses the AP-DRG system as its base. It also uses two other measures to assign patients to categories that include mortality risk and severity of illness factors, assigning patients to subclasses that identify minor, moderate, major, or extreme severity of illness or risk of mortality.

Case-Mix Index

The case-mix index for a hospital is defined as the average MS-DRG weight for all patients over a specified time period. A high case-mix index would signify that the patients treated in the facility were, on average, sicker than those in facilities with a lower case-mix index.

Other Uses of MS-DRGs

Although MS-DRGs are primarily used for payment, the hospital can use the data for many other purposes. One of those is for utilization review. By examining the MS-DRG data, the facility can examine utilization patterns among similar groups of patients to study variances and problem areas. Hospitals can review differences among physicians to determine reasons for variations in practice patterns or overutilization of ancillary services. Reports can be generated, such as top ten MS-DRGs, which can provide data that can be reviewed to determine appropriateness of services or provide topics for auditing.

Financial services can use the data for hospital cost analysis with up-to-date information on MS-DRGs for patients being discharged and the costs for treating these patients. Revenue can be monitored in a timely fashion to detect potential problems. Additionally, data can be used to help plan for new services, such as determining whether the facility should expand certain services. Moreover, they can be used for benchmarking best practices with other, similar facilities for epidemiology studies and research. As discussed in chapter 1, Medicare and other

Table 3.5. Examples of comparisons between DRG and MS-DRG systems

FY08 MS-DRG V25	FY08 MS-DRG Descriptions	FY08 Weight	FY08 1=Txfer 2=Spl Pay	FY07 CMS DRG V24	FY07 CMS V24 DRG Description	FY07 Weight	FY07 1=Txfer DRG 2=Spl Pay
177	Respiratory infections & inflammations w MCC	1.8444	1	079	Respiratory infections & inflammations age greater 17 w/ CC	1.6268	1
178	Respiratory infections & inflammations w CC	1.5636	1	080	Respiratory infections & inflammations age greater 17 w/o CC	0.8943	1
179	Respiratory infections & inflammations w/o CC/MCC	1.2754	1	081	Respiratory infections & inflammations age 0-17	1.5579	
180	Respiratory neoplasms w MCC	1.5550		082	Respiratory neoplasm	1.4121	1
181	Respiratory neoplasms w CC	1.3126					
182	Respiratory neoplasms w/o CC/MCC	1.1455					
183	Major chest trauma w MCC	1.2664		083	Major chest trauma w CC	1.0308	1
184	Major chest trauma w CC	0.9611		084	Major chest trauma w/o CC	0.6028	1
185	Major chest trauma w/o CC/MCC	0.7298					
186	Pleural effusion w MCC	1.4542	1	085	Pleural effusion w/ CC	1.2459	1
187	Pleural effusion w CC	1.1947	1	086	Pleural effusion w/o CC	0.7132	1
188	Pleural effusion w/o CC/MCC	0.9745	1				
189	Pulmonary edema & respiratory failure	1.3660		087	Pulmonary edema & respiratory failure	1.3838	
190	Chronic obstructive pulmonary disease w MCC	1.1138	1	088	Chronic obstructive pulmonary disease	0.8878	
191	Chronic obstructive pulmonary disease w CC	0.9405	1				
192	Chronic obstructive pulmonary disease w/o CC/MCC	0.8145	1				
193	Simple pneumonia & pleurisy w MCC	1.2505	1	089	Simple pneumonia & pleurisy age greater 17 w/ CC	1.0376	1
194	Simple pneumonia & pleurisy w CC	1.0235	1	090	Simple pneumonia & pleurisy age greater 17 w/o CC	0.6148	1
195	Simple pneumonia & pleurisy w/o CC/MCC	0.8398	1	091	Simple pneumonia age 0-17	0.5598	
196	Interstitial lung disease w MCC	1.3781	1	092	Interstitial lung disease w/ CC	1.1979	1
197	Interstitial lung disease w CC	1.1458	1	093	Interstitial lung disease w/o CC	0.7437	1
198	Interstitial lung disease w/o CC/MCC	0.9654	1				
199	Pneumothorax w MCC	1.4699		094	Pneumothorax w/ CC	1.1474	
200	Pneumothorax w CC	1.0753		095	Pneumothorax w/o CC	0.5871	
201	Pneumothorax w/o CC/MCC	0.8588					
202	Bronchitis & asthma w CC/MCC	0.7841		096	Bronchitis & asthma age greater 17 w/ CC	0.7350	
203	Bronchitis & asthma w/o CC/MCC	0.6252		097	Bronchitis & asthma age greater 17 w/o CC	0.5429	
				098	Bronchitis & asthma age 0-17	0.5870	
204	Respiratory signs & symptoms	0.6658		099	Respiratory signs and symptoms w/ CC	0.7155	
				100	Respiratory signs and symptoms w/o CC	0.5411	

Table available at CMS website: www.cms.hhs.gov/Medicare/Acute
Inpatient PPS/Acute Inpatient—Files for Download Crosswalk for CMS DRGs to MS-DRGs
Table 5 FY08 and Table 5 FY07 lists DRG weights

Source: Spencer and Hyde 2008, appendix B, 68.

third party payers are utilizing pay-for-performance quality incentives to tie reimbursement to quality of care. The data obtained during MS-DRG assignment is used in part to enable facilities to meet reporting requirements.

Summary

The DRG payment system, which has been in place now for approximately twenty-seven years, just changed to MS-DRGs and is used by Medicare to pay for hospital inpatient admissions. Each year, as the system is updated, it attempts to accurately reflect appropriate payment necessary to treat the changing Medicare population. Medicare is moving ahead in its plans to capture more severity of illness information on the Medicare population. The adoption of the MS-DRG system update has brought major changes to this payment system, so coders should familiarize themselves with these updates and various alternatives also being discussed and used by other insurance companies to pay for hospital inpatient care.

Chapter 4

Structure and Organization of Other Medicare Inpatient Prospective Payment Systems

Because the federal government considered diagnosis-related groups (DRGs) to be helpful in managing costs and resource consumption in the acute care hospital inpatient setting, over the years legislation has been passed that requires prospective payment–type systems in other healthcare settings. This chapter discusses some of the Medicare systems in place for reimbursement in inpatient settings other than acute care hospitals. These include long-term acute care hospitals, inpatient rehabilitation hospitals, and inpatient psychiatric facilities.

Long-Term Care Prospective Payment System

The Balanced Budget Refinement Act of 1999 and the Benefits Improvement and Protection Act of 2000 established the requirements for a prospective payment system (PPS) for long-term acute care hospitals (LTCHs), effective with discharges on or after October 1, 2002. Medicare defines LTCHs as hospitals that (CMS 2004):

> . . . have an average inpatient length of stay greater than 25 days. These hospitals typically provide extended medical and rehabilitative care for patients who are clinically complex and may suffer from multiple acute or chronic conditions. Services may include comprehensive rehabilitation, respiratory therapy, cancer treatment, head trauma treatment, and pain management.

The long-term care hospital prospective payment system (LTCH PPS) is based on the inpatient PPS (IPPS) system with modifications made to account for differences in the long-term care patient and was started in 2003. When Medicare updated the Medicare Severity Adjusted diagnosis-related groups (MS-DRG) system in FY 2008, the long-term care DRG system was also updated to a modified MS-DRG system. There are also special rules covering occurrences such as short stays, very-high-cost admissions, and interrupted stays. This system was put into place in October 2003. Patients' stays are grouped into categories known as Medicare Severity-adjusted Long-term Care Hospital Diagnosis Related Groups (MS-LTC-DRGs), based on their diagnoses, procedures performed and discharge status. Like the inpatient MS-DRG system, the MS-LTC-DRG grouping (CMS 2006b):

> . . . reflects the differences in patient resources and costs in LTCHs while maintaining budget neutrality and reflects the typical resources used for treating such a patient.

Also like the DRG System, the MS-LTC-DRG system was designed to pay only one amount of reimbursement per hospitalization, which is assigned at discharge.

Coders must follow the same rules as those used for coding IPPSs, which includes following Official Coding Guidelines and the UHDDS definitions. This includes the definition for principal diagnosis, complications, comorbidities, those conditions that affect treatment, and all procedures performed during the patient's stay. The same grouper software is used for calculating MS-LTC-DRG as is used for inpatient DRG grouping with relative weights that are reflective of patients in the long-term acute care setting. Payment rates are based on data in the MedPar database consisting of claims previously submitted by LTCHs.

The major elements of the long-term care hospital PPS are described in the following sections.

Patient Classification System

Patients are grouped into DRG-type groupings based on the clinical aspects of their disease as well as the amount of resources needed for their care.

Relative Weights

Each MS-LTC-DRG is weighted, as with the IPPS weights, to reflect patients treated in LTCH-type settings.

Rate of Payment

Similar to the IPPS, facility payment is based on a set fee per discharge that takes into account the resources used to care for the patient. Adjustments are made for short-stay cases, interrupted stays, readmissions within a certain time frame, cost outliers, and geographic wage rate and cost of living increases. Updates are made annually.

Interrupted Stays

Interrupted-stay cases are those cases in which patients have an "intervening" stay during the time of their long-term care admission. When a patient is admitted as an inpatient in an acute care hospital for 9 or fewer days, an inpatient rehabilitation facility for 27 or fewer days, or a skilled nursing facility for 45 or fewer days, and the time of the interruption is three or fewer days, the two long-term care stays are paid as one stay. According to the LTCH interrupted-stay fact sheet (CMS 2008b, 2):

> If the interruption exceeds 3 days, LTCH payment will be determined under the original interrupted stay policy (referred to as a "greater than 3-day interruption of stay"), but the day count for purposes of determining the length of the stay away from the LTCH begins on the day that the patient is first discharged from the LTCH. Medicare payment for any test, procedure, or care provided to the patient on either an outpatient or inpatient basis during the "interruption" would be the responsibility of the LTCH "under arrangements."

Short-Stay Outliers

Cases where the length of stay (LOS) is between one day and up to or equal to or less than five-sixths of the average LOS for the respective MS-LTC-DRG are considered short-stay outliers. Medicare also removes cases with an LOS of seven or fewer days from statistical formulas when setting MS-LTC-DRG relative weights because these stays alter the law-of-averages principle on which the DRG system was built (CMS 2008c).

Hospital-Specific Relative Value Method

Because various LTCHs tend to treat different groups of patients, the Centers for Medicare and Medicaid Services (CMS) developed an adjustment method known as the hospital-specific relative value method. This method converts charges for each LTCH into hospital-specific values that then are adjusted based on the individual hospital's case mix.

Transition Period

A five-year transition period was implemented on October 1, 2002, to phase in the PPS for LTCHs from cost-based reimbursement to 100 percent federal prospective payment. Payment was based on an increasing percentage of the LTCH PPS amount and a decreasing percentage of the cost-based reimbursement rate for each discharge. This phase-in period was typical of that used with the other types of prospective payment methods to prevent undue financial hardship on facilities in the early days of the new systems. According to CMS (2007e, 24823), "for cost reporting periods beginning on or after October 1, 2006, all LTCHs are paid 100 percent of the adjusted federal rate under the LTCH PPS."

The fiscal year, or rate year (RY), was set to begin on July 1 each year and end on June 30, which requires two updates per year. In July, the federal rate is updated and in October the MS-LTC-DRG and weights are updated to incorporate the annual October 1 ICD-9-CM and IPPS changes. Although ICD-9-CM codes may be updated twice per year, the groupings and relative weights established in the MS-LTC-DRG system are updated only in October. See table 4.1 for a portion of the MS-LTC-DRG list. Additional information on MS-LTC-DRGs is available from CMS' long-term care hospital PPS overview (2006b).

Inpatient Rehabilitation Hospital Prospective Payment System

Implementation of a per discharge PPS for inpatient rehabilitation facilities (IRFs) was authorized in section 4421 of the Balanced Budget Act of 1997 (Public Law 105-33), as amended by section 125 of the Medicare, Medicaid, and State Children's Health Insurance Program (SCHIP) Balanced Budget Refinement Act of 1999 (Public Law 106-113), and by section 305 of the Medicare, Medicaid, and SCHIP Benefits Improvement and Protection Act of 2000 (Public Law 106-554), authorized through new section 1886(j) of the Social Security Act (CMS 2007g).

In 1995, CMS sponsored a study by the RAND Corporation to develop an IRF per discharge PPS using a system known as functional independence measures–functional-related groups (FIM-FRGs). This study was updated in 1999 to reflect payment information, including facility payment adjustments and the impact of other diagnoses (comorbidities) on patient resource utilization.

To account for the types of patients treated in IRFs, this system uses information from the patient assessment instrument (PAI). The information from the resulting IRF patient assessment instrument (IRF-PAI) is entered electronically into grouper software, which determines the health insurance prospective payment system (HIPPS) codes used to establish reimbursement. The software is known as Inpatient Rehabilitation Validation and Entry (IRVEN) and is provided at no cost to facilities (CMS 2007h).

The HIPPS codes then are grouped into one of 100 case-mix groups, which determines reimbursement for the hospitalization.

Table 4.1. Portion of the MS-LTC-DRG list

MS-LTC-DRG	MS-DRG Title	FY 2006 LTCH Cases	FY 2008 Relative Weight	Geometric Average Length of Stay	Short Stay Outlier Threshold	IPPS Comparable Threshold
1	Heart transplant or implant of heart assist system w MCC	0	0.0000	0.0	0.0	0.0
2	Heart transplant or implant of heart assist system w/o MCC	0	0.0000	0.0	0.0	0.0
3	ECMO or trach w MV 96+ hrs or PDX exc face, mouth & neck w maj O.R.	280	4.2380	64.3	53.6	53.6
4	Trach w MV 96+ hrs or PDX exc face, mouth & neck w/o maj O.R.	1067	3.0249	46.7	38.9	38.9
5	Liver transplant w MCC or intestinal transplant	0	0.0000	0.0	0.0	0.0
6	Liver transplant w/o MCC	0	0.0000	0.0	0.0	0.0
7	Lung transplant	0	0.0000	0.0	0.0	0.0
8	Simultaneous pancreas/ kidney transplant	0	0.0000	0.0	0.0	0.0
9	Bone marrow transplant	0	1.1417	29.0	24.2	24.2
10	Pancreas transplant	0	0.0000	0.0	0.0	0.0
11	Tracheostomy for face, mouth & neck diagnoses w MCC	0	1.5545	35.2	29.3	25.2
12	Tracheostomy for face, mouth & neck diagnoses w CC	1	1.5545	35.2	29.3	16.7
13	Tracheostomy for face, mouth & neck diagnoses w/o CC/MCC	0	1.5545	35.2	29.3	11.2
20	Intracranial vascular procedures w PDX hemorrhage w MCC	0	1.5545	35.2	29.3	29.3
21	Intracranial vascular procedures w PDX hemorrhage w CC	0	0.5472	20.3	16.9	16.9
22	Intracranial vascular procedures w PDX hemorrhage w/o CC/MCC	0	0.5472	20.3	16.9	16.1
23	Cranio w major dev impl/ acute complex CNS PDX w MCC or chemo implant	0	1.5545	35.2	29.3	22.2

Source: CMS 2007f.

Rehabilitation Impairment Categories

Prior to placing the patient in one of the case-mix groups, the patient is grouped into a major group reflective of the primary need for rehabilitation care, which is known as the rehabilitation impairment category (RIC). Currently, there are twenty-one RICs in use in the IRF PPS system, as listed in figure 4.1. Within each RIC, there are several case-mix groups based on established criteria, such as patients' ability to care for themselves and age. CMS used a statistical method to effectively group the patients into the case-mix groups based on a method known as classification and regression trees (CART).

Case-Mix Groups

The case-mix groups (CMG) consist of five-digit numbers. The first digit represents the comorbidity tier and the last four digits represent the actual case-mix grouping. Table 4.2 provides a sample of current CMGs.

Figure 4.1. List of RICs for IRFs

1. Stroke	13. Rheumatoid, Other Arthritis
2. Traumatic Brain Injury	14. Cardiac
3. Nontraumatic Brain Injury	15. Pulmonary
4. Traumatic Spinal Cord Injury	16. Pain Syndrome
5. Nontraumatic Spinal Cord Injury	17. Major multiple trauma, no brain injury or spinal cord injury
6. Neurological	
7. Fracture of Lower Extremity	18. Major multiple trauma, with brain or spinal cord injury
8. Replacement of Lower Extremity Joint	
9. Other Orthopedic	19. Guillain Barre
10. Amputation, Lower Extremity	20. Miscellaneous
11. Amputation, Other	21. Burns
12. Osteoarthritis	

Table 4.2. Relative weights and average LOS for CMGs

CMG	CMG Description (M = Motor, C = Cognitive, A = Age)	Relative Weights				Average Length of Stay			
		Tier 1	Tier 2	Tier 3	None	Tier 1	Tier 2	Tier 3	None
0101	Stroke M > 51.05	0.7707	0.7303	0.6572	0.6347	8	11	9	9
0102	Stroke M > 44.45 and M < 51.05 and C > 18.5	0.9493	0.8995	0.8095	0.7818	11	15	11	10
0103	Stroke M > 44.45 and M < 51.05 and C < 18.5	1.1192	1.0605	0.9544	0.9218	14	13	12	12
0104	Stroke M > 38.85 and M < 44.45	1.1885	1.1260	1.0134	0.9787	13	14	13	13
0105	Stroke M > 34.25 and M < 38.85	1.4261	1.3512	1.2161	1.1745	16	17	16	15

Source: CMS 2007g, 44293.

Comorbidities

Comorbidities are secondary diagnoses the patient has in conjunction with his or her primary illness or injury. The presence of these comorbidities may have an impact on the patient's rate of recovery, so when the IRF system was developed, the comorbidities were accounted for in the relative weight of each case-mix group. Just as in the other PPS systems, the relative weights help to differentiate between resources required to care for patients within the case-mix group. For instance, a weight of 2 means that, on average, it takes twice as many resources to care for patients than it would in a category with a weight of 1.

The "comorbidity tier" represents comorbid conditions that have been shown statistically to increase the amount of resources consumed by the patient. For example, a diagnosis of acute myocardial infarction adds cost to the patient's care, so the facility is entitled to greater reimbursement. Some procedures, such as dialysis, also increase the costs associated with the patient's care, so patients undergoing those procedures are placed in tier one.

Case-mix groups were designed using criteria including age, functional status, and rehabilitation impairment categories. Patients are assigned to a case-mix group based on their ability to function in categories such as transfer, self-care, sphincter control, and movement, as well as thirteen motor tasks and five cognitive tasks. New data added to the IRF-PAI also include items such as shortness of breath and presence of ulcers. According to instructions in the *CMS IRF-PAI Instruction Manual,* the cognitive and motor skills are evaluated and assigned a score from 0 to 7, with 7 meaning that the patient is very comfortable in performing the skill (2004b). A score of 0 means the skill cannot or did not occur. For payment purposes, a 0 is changed to a 1 to show that the patient requires total assistance in order to complete the task. Beginning in FY 2006, the motor skills scores were weighted based on the average ability of patients to perform the functions identified. See figure 4.2 for the motor and cognitive tasks that are evaluated to assess patients' functional status.

Five case-mix groups were designed to capture data on patients who died while in an IRF as well as patients whose stays were relatively short compared to most IRF patients. Each case-mix group was weighted to account for variation in resource consumption across the IRF patient spectrum, as well as the impact of additional (comorbid) diseases. Additionally, adjustments were made for a facility with a high percentage of low-income patients, wage variations, and rural location, as well as transfers, interrupted stays, and cost outliers (CMS 2007i). A new adjustment for teaching facilities was added in 2005. Table 4.3 presents the special case-mix groups not included in the RIC categories.

Qualification as an IRF

To qualify as an IRF, 75 percent of the patients treated must fall into medical conditions listed in figure 4.3.

Figure 4.2.   Motor and cognitive tasks assessed on the IRF-PAI

Eating	Walking/wheelchair use
Grooming	Climbing stairs
Bathing	Cognitive skills:
Dressing upper body	Social interaction
Dressing lower body	Expression
Toileting	Memory
Bladder and bowel management	Comprehension
Transfer to:	Problem solving
Tub/shower, toilet, bed/chair/wheelchair	

Table 4.3.   Special case-mix groups not included in the RIC categories

CMG	Description
5001	Short-stay cases, LOS 3 days or less
5101	Expired, Orthopedic, LOS 13 days or less
5102	Expired, Orthopedic, LOS 14 days or more
5103	Expired, Not Orthopedic, LOS 15 days or less
5104	Expired, Not Orthopedic, LOS 16 days or more

Source: CMS 2007g, 44297.

Figure 4.3.   IRF medical condition qualifier

- Stroke
- Spinal cord injury
- Congenital deformity
- Amputation
- Major multiple trauma
- Femur fracture (hip fracture)
- Brain injury
- Neurological disorders, including multiple sclerosis, motor neuron diseases, polyneuropathy, muscular dystrophy, and Parkinson's disease
- Burns
- Active polyarticular rheumatoid arthritis, psoriatic arthritis, and seronegative arthropathies resulting in significant functional impairment of ambulation and other activities of daily living that have not improved after an appropriate, aggressive, and sustained course of outpatient therapy services or services in other, less intensive rehabilitation settings immediately preceding the inpatient rehabilitation admission or that result from a systemic disease activation immediately before admission but have the potential to improve with more intense rehabilitation
- Systemic vasculidities with joint inflammation arthropathies resulting in significant functional impairment of ambulation and other activities of daily living that have not improved after an appropriate, aggressive, and sustained course of outpatient therapy services or services in other, less intensive rehabilitation settings immediately preceding the inpatient rehabilitation admission or that result from a systemic disease activation immediately before admission but have the potential to improve with more intense rehabilitation
- Severe or advanced osteoarthritis (osteoarthrosis or degenerative joint disease) involving two or more major weight-bearing joints (elbows, shoulders, hips, or knees, but not counting a joint with a prosthesis) with joint deformity and substantial loss of range of motion, atrophy of muscles surrounding the joint, significant functional impairment of ambulation and other activities of daily living that have not improved after an appropriate, aggressive, and sustained course of outpatient therapy services or services in other, less intensive rehabilitation settings immediately preceding the inpatient rehabilitation admission or that result from a systemic disease activation immediately before admission but have the potential to improve with more intense rehabilitation. (A joint replaced by a prosthesis is no longer considered to have osteoarthritis or other arthritis, even though this condition was the reason for the replacement.)
- Knee or hip joint replacement, or both, during an acute hospitalization immediately preceding the hospital rehabilitation stay, which also meet one or more of the following specific criteria:
  —The patient underwent bilateral knee or bilateral hip joint replacement surgery during the acute hospital admission immediately preceding the IRF admission.
  —The patient is extremely obese with a body mass index of at least 50 at the time of admission to the IRF.
  —The patient is age 85 or older at the time of admission to the IRF

Source: CMS 2007i, appendix A, 13.

To count in the IRF's percentage rate, the patient must have had an acute hospitalization for the condition and documented evidence must show that the patient failed a less aggressive treatment (at least twice per week) for a three-week period within 20 days following admission. If a facility fails to meet the requirements during a 12-month period, the hospital will lose certification as an IRF and will be paid under the methodology for an acute care facility.

Prior to July 1, 2008, patients who have the conditions listed in figure 4.3 as either their principal or secondary diagnoses will count in the percentage rate. After July 1, 2008, the condition must be the first-listed principal diagnosis (main reason for the admission) or the patient will not be counted in the overall percentage rate.

Inpatient Psychiatric Facilities

The Balanced Budget Refinement Act of 1999 required that a PPS be established for licensed inpatient psychiatric hospitals and hospital-based psychiatric units. This inpatient psychiatric facility (IPF) PPS was to be phased in over a three-year period starting with discharges on or after January 1, 2005. For cost reporting periods beginning on or after January 1, 2008, all IPFs will be paid 100 percent of the federal per diem payment amount (CMS 2007d, 47136). Like most of the other PPS systems, this system is based on the inpatient DRG system with modifications to account for differences unique to the patients needing intensive psychiatric treatment. Updates to the IPF PPS are effective on July 1 of each year to allow for a yearly cycle to begin in July.

IPF Coding

Although psychiatric facilities are accustomed to using the *Diagnostic and Statistical Manual of Mental Disorders, Fourth Edition* (DSM-IV) coding system, the PPS is based on codes found in ICD-9-CM (CMS 2007k, 25609).

Facilities are required to use the definition of principal diagnosis for selection of the first code to list on the billing form. IPF facilities also may code up to eight additional diagnosis codes as well as one principal procedure code and up to five additional procedure codes.

IPF Payment Adjustments

Like most of the PPS systems, Medicare has included a stop-loss provision that keeps the hospitals from having to sustain large losses in funds as they transition into the new system. The IPF system consists of a per diem (per day) payment. Beginning on January 1, 2008, the stop loss period ended and payments are based 100 percent on the IRF PPS payment rates.

CMS also has allowed for adjustments to account for patients receiving electroconvulsive therapy and interrupted stays and adjustments for teaching facilities, wage index variations, and payments to facilities in rural areas. A facility with a fully functioning emergency department receives an additional adjustment for the first day of treatment as well.

DRG-Specific Adjustments

The inpatient DRG system is used to group IPF patients into fifteen psychiatric DRG categories, although the inpatient payment methodology is not used in the psychiatric payment system. When a patient has a principal diagnosis found in one of the fifteen specified psychiatric DRGs, the IPF receives an additional amount above the federal per diem base rate. (See table 4.4 for a list of psychiatric DRGs.)

Table 4.4.   Psychiatric DRGs

Types of DRGs	DRG Code	Adjustment Factors
Procedure w principal diagnosis of mental illness	DRG 424	1.22
Acute adjustment reaction	DRG 425	1.05
Depressive neurosis	DRG 426	0.99
Neurosis, except depressive	DRG 427	1.02
Disorders of personality	DRG 428	1.02
Organic disturbances	DRG 429	1.03
Psychosis	DRG 430	1.00
Childhood disorders	DRG 431	0.99
Other mental disorders	DRG 432	0.92
Alcohol/Drug use, LAMA	DRG 433	0.97
Alcohol/Drug, w CC	DRG 521	1.02
Alcohol/Drug, w/o CC	DRG 522	0.98
Alcohol/Drug use, w/o rehab	DRG 523	0.88
Degenerative nervous system disorders	DRG 12	1.05
Non-traumatic stupor & coma	DRG 23	1.07

Source: CMS 2007k.

Comorbidities are those secondary conditions that affect the patient's ability to recover and benefit from treatment. Seventeen groups of comorbid conditions generate an additional payment under the IPF PPS system. Table 4.5 shows the comorbidity groupings.

Finally, nine age group adjustments are made for patients aged 45 years and older, as listed in table 4.6.

Electroconvulsive Therapy

When patients receive electroconvulsive therapy (ECT) during an IPF admission, the facility should bill ICD-9-CM code 94.27 under revenue code 0901 to receive the additional payment. The total number of ECT treatments received should be indicated in the "service units" category on the same line item on the bill.

Interrupted Stays

Inpatients who have to be transferred to other types of facilities for treatment not performed in the IPF facility, such as dialysis, are still considered inpatients. However, when the patient is discharged and readmitted to the same or another IPF prior to midnight on the third day (that is, the length of the interruption is three or fewer days), the IPF stay is paid as one episode of care rather than two. When the patient is not officially discharged, the IPF retains responsibility for care during the interruption. This policy was developed to prevent facilities from discharging

Table 4.5.   IPF PPS cormorbidity groupings

Description of Comorbidity	Code	Adjustment
Developmental Disabilities	317, 318.0, 318.1, 318.2, and 319	1.04
Coagulation Factor Deficits	2860 through 2864	1.13
Tracheotomy	51900 through 51909 and V440	1.06
Renal Failure, Acute	5845 through 5849, 6363, 6373, 6383, 6393, 66932, 66934, 9585	1.11
Renal Failure, Chronic	40301, 40311, 40391, 40402, 40403, 40412, 40413, 40492, 40493, 585, 586, V451, V560, V561, and V562	1.11
Oncology Treatment	1400 through 2399 WITH either V58.0 OR V58.1	1.07
Uncontrolled Type I Diabetes Mellitus, with or without complications	25002, 25003, 25012, 25013, 25022, 25023, 25032, 25033, 25042, 25043, 25052, 25053, 25062, 25063, 25072, 25073, 25082, 25083, 25092, and 25093	1.05
Severe Protein Calorie Malnutrition	260 through 262	1.13
Eating and Conduct Disorders	3071, 30750, 31203, 31233, and 31234	1.12
Infectious Disease	01000 through 04110, 042, 04500 through 05319, 05440 through 05449, 0550 through 0770, 0782 through 07889, and 07950 through 07959	1.07
Drug and/or Alcohol Induced Mental Disorders	2910, 2920, 2922, 30300, and 30400	1.03
Cardiac Conditions	3910, 3911, 3912, 40201, 40403, 4160, 4210, 4211, and 4219	1.11
Gangrene	44024 and 7854	1.10
Chronic Obstructive Pulmonary Disease	49121, 4941, 5100, 51883, 51884, and V461	1.12
Artificial Openings—Digestive and Urinary	56960 through 56969, 9975, and V441 through V446	1.08
Severe Musculoskeletal and Connective Tissue Diseases	6960, 7100, 73000 through 73009, 73010 through 73019, and 73020 through 73029	1.09
Poisoning	96500 through 96509, 9654, 9670 through 9699, 9770, 9800 through 9809, 9830 through 9839, 986, 9890 through 9897	1.11

Source: CMS 2007k, 25610.

Table 4.6. Age groupings and adjustment factors

Age	Adjustment Factor
Under 45	1.00
45 and under 50	1.01
50 and under 55	1.02
55 and under 60	1.04
60 and under 65	1.07
65 and under 70	1.10
70 and under 75	1.13
75 and under 80	1.15
80 and over	1.17

Source: CMS 2007k, 25613–25614.

and readmitting patients to receive the higher per diem rate associated with the early days of new admissions. CMS has instructed IPFs to hold claims for three days to check for readmissions prior to billing (CMS 2007k).

Other Adjustments

Teaching facilities receive an adjustment based on the ratio of interns and residents as compared to the average daily census. There is also an outlier payment policy. When the patient's costs exceed a fixed amount, CMS shares in additional costs based on the number of days the patient is treated in the facility.

Summary

Prospective payment systems have been adapted successfully for a number of inpatient settings other than acute short term care hospitals. Long-term care facilities, inpatient rehabilitation hospitals, and inpatient psychiatric facilities all operate today under unique prospective payment requirements and modifications.

Part II

Coding for Inpatient Services

Chapter 5

Diagnostic and Procedural Coding for Inpatient Services

Clinical coding, the process of transforming verbal descriptions of diseases, injuries, conditions, and procedures into numerical designations, has been a health information management (HIM) function since the health record profession was established. It has enabled healthcare facilities and associated agencies to tabulate, store, and retrieve disease-, injury-, and procedure-related data. With the passage of numerous pieces of legislation over the years that have required code assignment as a condition for reimbursement, coding has taken on increased significance.

Under prospective payment systems, coding is linked directly to the healthcare facility's financial viability, and ICD-9-CM codes are the primary element of many of the prospective payment systems (PPSs). Billing cannot be done until documentation is sufficient to allow for complete coding.

The inpatient PPS marked the beginning of a new era for the health information service and the update of the system to account for severity of illness has yet again brought the coding process under increased scrutiny. As more healthcare areas have migrated to some form of prospective payment, the need for effectively managing coded data has increased and there is a high demand for the expertise of credentialed coding professionals. Coded information is reported to state and national databases and used for facility report cards, quality reporting, and benchmarking. As stated in *Top 200 Coding Hospitals* (Ingenix 2007):

> The health care industry's increasing reliance on code-based prospective payment systems, such as diagnosis-related groups and ambulatory payment classifications, underscores the critical impact of clinical documentation and coding on hospital revenues. The primary purpose is to use data to benchmark coding performance, improve revenue management and quality reporting.

This chapter discusses general coding rules and guidelines and how they are implemented in facility coding policies.

Ethical Coding

As health information services face the pressures of deadlines and outside review agencies, adoption of ethical practice standards becomes increasingly important. Recognizing the increased responsibility of coding professionals, the board of directors of the American

Health Information Management Association (AHIMA) developed a Code of Ethics. (See appendix A, pp. 149–157.) The Code of Ethics is intended to serve as a guide to ethical practice for coders and health information services by which departmental coding practices can be measured.

Coding Conventions, Rules, and Guidelines

Although many rules are involved in the coding process, in some cases, code selection is based on several different sets of rules within the coding hierarchy. Coders first must understand and utilize the rules in the ICD-9-CM coding book. This includes following all sequencing and cross-reference instructions found in the book. For example, when a patient has the diagnosis of diabetic retinopathy, the coder would find the following notations:

> **Retinopathy**
> Diabetic 250.5 *[362.01]*

When ICD-9-CM shows two codes listed in such a fashion, the coder should assign both codes to fully identify the patient's condition and must list them in the order in which they are printed in the book. In other words, the book is giving a sequencing rule: code the underlying disease (in this case, the diabetes [250.5x]) first, followed by the code for the manifestation (the retinopathy [362.01]). Manifestation codes are printed in italics and can never be sequenced as the first-listed diagnosis nor may they stand alone as a diagnosis. All other sequencing rules are superseded by this codebook instruction. After following the code book rules, the coding professional must adhere to any Official Coding Guidelines, and third in the hierarchy includes the official guidance provided in the *Coding Clinic* for ICD-9-CM.

The Cooperating Parties

The four agencies that have responsibility for maintaining and updating the ICD-9-CM coding system are known as the Cooperating Parties. These agencies are:

- The American Hospital Association (AHA), which maintains the Central Office on ICD-9-CM to answer case specific questions from coders and publishes the *Coding Clinic for ICD-9-CM* (1991–2008).

- The National Center for Health Statistics (NCHS), a branch of the Centers for Disease Control and Prevention, which maintains and updates the diagnosis portion of ICD-9-CM (Volumes 1 and 2) and releases the *ICD-9-CM Official Guidelines for Coding and Reporting,* available on its Web site (2007).

- The Centers for Medicare and Medicaid Services (CMS), which maintains and updates the procedure portion of ICD-9-CM, Volume 3 (n.d.).

- The American Health Information Management Association (AHIMA), which provides training and coding resources and certifications for coding professionals (2008a, 2008b).

The Cooperating parties' Web sites are included in the reference list (pp. 221–224).

ICD-9-CM Official Guidelines for Coding and Reporting

One of the main duties of the Cooperating Parties is to develop the official coding guidelines to provide detailed and official rules for the use of ICD-9-CM coding.

Health Insurance Portability and Accountability Act of 1996

In 2000, the Department of Health and Human Services (HHS) set forth regulations for electronic transactions and coding standards as mandated by the Health Insurance Portability and Accountability Act (HIPAA) of 1996. HIPAA designated ICD-9-CM diagnosis codes as the official standard for coding diagnoses in all facilities and ICD-9-CM procedure codes as the standard for coding procedures for hospital inpatients. The ICD-9-CM Official Guidelines for Coding and Reporting also were named in the rulings, establishing that in order to be in compliance with HIPAA, all entities must utilize and follow the official guidelines (Schraffenberger and Kuehn 2007, 14).

Many publishers have included references to specific official coding guidelines in their coding publications.

Coding Clinic for ICD-9-CM

Coding Clinic for ICD-9-CM is a quarterly publication of AHA. According to the September 3, 1986, *Federal Register* (as quoted in AHIMA 2008):

> Coding guidelines are clarified through unanimous agreement by the cooperating parties, and the primary role of the cooperating parties is to approve the contents of each issue of *Coding Clinic for ICD-9-CM.*

The Cooperating Parties achieve this by serving as the only voting members of the editorial advisory board of *Coding Clinic for ICD-9-CM. Coding Clinic* addresses questions from across the country and publishes official coding advice and includes the ICD-9-CM Guidelines for Coding and Reporting in their publication. The Editorial Review Board, made up of members representing the Cooperating Parties, review articles, responses to questions, and answers in *Coding Clinic* prior to publication. The advice given is to be followed by coders in all settings, including physician office, clinic, outpatient, and hospital inpatient coding. Coders should review this publication regularly for updated information regarding ICD-9-CM coding.

ICD-9-CM Coordination and Maintenance Committee

In 1985, the ICD-9-CM Coordination and Maintenance Committee was established to provide a public forum for discussion of revisions to the *International Classification of Diseases, 9th Revision, Clinical Modification* (ICD-9-CM) codebook. This federal committee is cochaired by representatives from NCHS and CMS and meets twice a year in Baltimore. Both the public and private sectors are encouraged to comment on the suggested modifications and to recommend changes to the ICD-9-CM codes. Decisions are not made at this meeting; however, comments are reviewed by the appropriate agency. The final modifications are published in the *Federal Register* and the *Official Authorized Addendum to the ICD-9-CM* (CDC 2008). Minutes and additional information can be obtained on the committee's Web site noted in the reference list (pp. 221–224).

Uniform Bill-04 (UB-04)

To standardize billing forms with the standardized systematized terminology required by the Uniform Hospital Data Discharge Set (UHDDS), the National Uniform Billing Committee (NUBC) developed Uniform Bill-82 (UB-82). This single, uniform bill consolidated the numerous forms that hospitals were using to submit bills to third-party payers. A revision of UB-82 was approved in 1992, and another revision became effective in March 2007. This revision, named UB-04, permits hospitals to report eighteen diagnosis codes and six procedure codes, although CMS only processes nine diagnosis codes and six procedure codes. UB-04 contains an admitting diagnosis field in addition to three fields for reason for visit on outpatient claims. Medicare and most other third-party payers require use of UB-04 for inpatient billing in hospitals. Although much of the data on the form are collected by the admission and financial services departments, the health information service supplies the clinical coded data that are placed on the form and must ensure their accuracy. Each state has a UB committee that incorporates specific requirements unique to that state.

The UB-04 billing form was also designed to accommodate changes brought about by new transaction standards for the electronic exchange of data and the eventual adoption of ICD-10-CM. The UB-04 form reflects increased emphasis now placed on the clinical coding components. More information on the UB-04 can be found on the NUBC Web site at www.nubc.org/new.html.

Coding Policies

Each hospital's health information service must identify its requirements for coded data and establish coding policies and procedures based on its health information needs. These should reflect the standard usage of the definitions as set forth by the UHDDS, the ICD-9-CM Official Guidelines for Coding and Reporting, and *Coding Clinic*, as overseen by the Cooperating Parties. Policies and procedures ensure that data is consistently reported for data analysis and reporting purposes. These requirements should be initiated by the director of the health information service in consultation with the administration, medical staff, and other healthcare professionals. Coded data may be needed for reimbursement, marketing, planning, utilization management, quality of care assessment, and research. New initiatives such as pay for performance, benchmarking, and quality reporting requirements are also based on coded data, so it is imperative that data is reported on a consistent basis.

At a minimum, coding policies should clarify how coding professionals should address issues such as the assignment of optional E codes and M code assignment "history of" diagnoses, not reporting incidental x-ray and laboratory findings, and informing which procedures should be coded by the coding professional. Facility-based coding guidelines should be developed for those areas that have not been addressed by the official sources for coding advice or that have been addressed but require expansion or definition for an individual facility. Policies should address the physician query process for coding clarification and how to handle inconsistent diagnoses by a single physician in chart documentation, as well as conflicting diagnoses among physicians. See appendix C (p. 173) for a sample physician query form. Some corporations have developed coding policies that are being used consistently by all the hospitals in their organizations.

Written coding policies may be helpful in resolving coding disputes with outside reviewers. However, such policies must adhere to UHDDS definitions and sequencing guidelines, as well as be applicable to ICD-9-CM coding principles and official ICD-9-CM coding guidelines.

Complete, accurate, and consistent coding of all diagnoses and procedures documented is required for compliant coding. The number of codes to be assigned depends on the statistical and retrieval needs of the health information service, including data needs for utilization management, quality management activities, hospital planning, research, pay for performance, and benchmarking. See appendix B (pp. 159–163) for AHIMA's practice brief on Developing a Coding Compliance Policy Document (2001). Sample coding policies are available online from HCA Management Services (1995–2004).

Uniform Hospital Discharge Data Set

In 1974, the Department of Health, Education, and Welfare developed what has become known as the Uniform Hospital Discharge Data Set (UHDDS.) The UHDDS is defined as (Schraffenberger and Kuehn 2007, 57):

> . . . a minimum, common core of data on individual acute care, short-term hospital discharges in Medicare and Medicaid programs. It sought to improve the uniformity and comparability of hospital discharge data.

Over the years, the definitions have been refined and updated as changes in healthcare continued. In its latest revision, it includes all "non-outpatient" settings, which include long-term acute care hospitals, psychiatric hospitals, home health agencies, and nursing homes. The prospective payment systems use the UHDDS definitions as the basis for making some payment decisions.

The UHDDS includes definitions for demographic information such as identification, race, and residence; encounter information such as admission and discharge dates, physician identification, and disposition of patient; and reimbursement information such as expected payer, diagnoses, and procedure definitions. With regard to prospective payment, the most important of these definitions include the definitions of principal diagnosis, selection of other diagnoses, and procedures.

Diagnoses

All diagnoses that affect the current hospital stay must be reported as part of the UHDDS. The *principal diagnosis* is designated and defined in the UHDDS as "the condition established after study to be chiefly responsible for occasioning the admission of the patient to the hospital for care" (NCVHS 1996). The words "after study" in this definition are most significant and cannot be ignored when selecting the principal diagnosis. Patients with symptoms that require further study before a definitive diagnosis can be identified are frequently admitted to hospitals. See table 5.1 for examples of such symptoms.

Other diagnoses are designated and defined as "all conditions that coexist at the time of admission, that develop subsequently, or that affect the treatment received and/or the length of stay" (NCVHS 1996). Diagnoses that relate to an earlier episode and that have no bearing on the current hospital stay are to be excluded. In addition, it is not appropriate for coding professionals to refer to previous admissions to obtain documentation to support coding of diagnoses for the current admission.

A *complication* is an *additional* diagnosis describing a condition arising after the beginning of hospital observation and treatment that modifies the course of the patient's illness or the medical care required. Complications prolong the patient's length of stay (LOS) by at least one day in 75 percent of cases. Progress notations by physicians, nurses, and other healthcare providers often describe signs and symptoms that represent possible complications. Before assigning a code, however, the coder should make sure that the attending physician has documented such notations appropriately and that there is no conflicting documentation found in the patient's health information. Examples of notations that provide possible clues to the actual condition are found in table 5.2.

Comorbidity is a preexisting condition that will, because of its presence with a specific principal diagnosis, cause an increase in the patient's LOS by at least one day in 75 percent of cases. Health record documentation must substantiate that the patient's management and care were affected by the conditions that coexisted at admission or that developed subsequently. In other words, the documentation should indicate that the patient received medication, other therapy, or diagnostic evaluation for each condition entered on the claim. For example, if diabetes mellitus is listed, the documentation should reflect either type I or type II diabetes and should also show that the patient was administered insulin or oral antidiabetics such as Diabinese, Orinase, or Tolinase. Additionally, the results of at least one blood glucose determination should be recorded. If a patient with type II diabetes receives insulin, the coder should also assign V58.67, long-term (current) use of insulin.

Table 5.1. Examples of symptoms requiring further study before a definitive diagnosis can be identified

Admitting Diagnosis	Diagnosis after Study
Severe abdominal pain	Diverticulitis with perforation
Severe abdominal pain	Ruptured ectopic pregnancy
Severe abdominal pain	Gastric ulcer with obstruction
Unexplained convulsions	Metastatic carcinoma of brain
Unexplained convulsions	Primary astrocytoma of brain
Unexplained convulsions	Convulsions NOS
Ascites	Cirrhosis of liver
Ascites	Metastatic carcinoma from breast to peritoneum with malignant ascites
Jaundice	Obstruction of common duct
Jaundice	Acute hepatitis A
Chest pain	Acute myocardial infarction
Chest pain	Gastroesophageal reflux disease

Table 5.2. Examples of notations that could indicate complicating conditions

Condition	Possible Clues
Wound disruption	Gaping postoperative wound with resuturing or other closure
Urinary tract infection	Symptoms of dysuria and frequency with orders for urine cultures
Myocardial infarction	Complaints of chest pain, orders for EKGs and cardiac enzyme/troponin studies

Principal Diagnosis Selection

The principal diagnosis is the key to appropriate reimbursement because it determines DRG assignment in most cases. However, errors in selecting the principal diagnosis are common.

At times, it seems that both physicians and coders have difficulty distinguishing between the principal diagnosis and the "most significant" diagnosis. The most significant diagnosis is the condition that has the most impact on the patient's health, LOS, and resource consumption. This diagnosis may or may not be the principal diagnosis. Each year, the OIG chooses problem prone areas to study and the hospital inpatient DRG system is always high on the list.

> **Example:** A patient is admitted with a fractured hip because of an accident. The fracture is reduced and the patient is discharged. After further study, the principal diagnosis is the fractured hip. If this same patient suffers a myocardial infarction during hospitalization, the myocardial infarction is a complication of the admission and should be coded as an additional diagnosis. The principal diagnosis remains the fractured hip.

In the example above, the myocardial infarction might be the most significant diagnosis in terms of the patient's health and resource consumption. After study, however, it is not found to be the reason for the patient's admission and thus is not the principal diagnosis.

Examples of continuous problem areas are discussed further in chapter 9.

Procedures and Date

All significant procedures must be reported. For significant procedures, the identity (by unique number within the hospital) of the person performing the procedure and the date the procedure was performed should be reported. Surgery includes incision, excision, amputation, introduction, endoscopy, repair, destruction, suture, and manipulation.

A *significant procedure* is one that:

- Is surgical in nature

- Carries a procedural risk

- Carries an anesthetic risk

- Requires specialized training

Procedural Risk

The term *procedural risk* refers to a professionally recognized risk that a given procedure may induce some functional impairment, injury, morbidity, or even death. This risk may arise from direct trauma, physiologic disturbances, interference with natural defense mechanisms, or exposure of the body to infection or other harmful agents. Traumatic procedures are those that are invasive (including nonsurgical procedures that use cutdowns), cause tissue damage (such as irradiation), or introduce some toxic or noxious substance (such as caustic test reagents).

Physiologic risk is associated with the use of virtually any pharmacologic or physical agent that can affect homeostasis (for example, those that alter fluid distribution, electrolyte balance, or blood pressure levels, and stress or tolerance tests).

Any procedure in which it is obligatory (or usual) to use pre- or postprocedure medications associated with physiologic or pharmacologic risk should be considered as having a procedural risk. For example, some procedures require heavy sedation using drugs selected for their systemic effects (such as alteration of metabolism, blood pressure, or cardiac function).

Some procedures may involve harmful exposures, such as cardiac catheterization, which may introduce bacteria into the bloodstream. Other procedures that carry an exposure risk include those capable of suppressing the immune system, those that can precipitate idiosyncratic reactions (such as anaphylaxis after the use of contrast materials), and those involving substances with known systemic toxicity (such as Digitoxin).

Long-life radioisotopes, such as carbon 14, pose a special kind of exposure risk to other persons as well as to the patient. These substances require special precautionary measures and the procedures for using them carry procedural risk.

Anesthetic Risk

Any procedure that requires or is regularly performed under general anesthesia carries anesthetic risk. This risk also occurs in procedures performed under local, regional, or other forms of anesthesia that induce sufficient functional impairment, necessitating special precautions to protect the patient from harm.

Specialized Training

This criterion is important for procedures that are performed exclusively or appropriately by specialized professionals, qualified technicians, or clinical teams either specifically trained for this purpose or whose services are dedicated principally to carrying them out. Whenever specially trained staff resources are necessary or are customarily employed in the performance of a procedure, it is considered significant.

Although procedural risks, anesthetic risk, and specialized training are defined in the UHDDS, it may be difficult for the coder to determine exactly which procedures require coding. Traditionally, however, healthcare facilities and third-party payers have not expected coders to code routine x-rays and laboratory tests. The coding policies of each hospital should be consulted to determine the procedures coded at that facility.

Principal Procedure

The term *principal procedure* is used for a procedure that was performed for definitive treatment, rather than one performed for diagnostic or exploratory purposes or to take care of a complication.

> **Example:** A patient admitted for hemoptysis undergoes a bronchoscopy with biopsy that reveals epidermoid carcinoma. Therefore, a left lower lobectomy is performed. The principal procedure is the left lower lobectomy because it was performed for definitive treatment; the bronchoscopy with biopsy was performed for diagnostic purposes.

When two procedures appear to be principal, the one most related to the principal diagnosis should be selected as the principal procedure.

> **Example:** Following an automobile accident, a patient was admitted with an open fracture of the neck of the femur, for which an open reduction with internal fixation was performed. During the hospitalization, the patient's

inguinal hernia became strangulated, requiring an inguinal herniorrhaphy to be performed. The reduction with internal fixation is the principal procedure because it is most related to the principal diagnosis of open fracture of the neck of the femur.

Many payers do not require that the principal procedure be sequenced first because they use computer software to select the highest-paying operative procedure. However, for correct data quality, it is important for the coder to select both the correct principal diagnosis and the correct principal procedure.

Medicare Code Editor

CMS provides Fiscal Intermediaries/Medicare Administrative Contractors (FI/MACs)with a Medicare Code Editor (MCE) to detect and report errors in the coding of claims data. This software is designed to detect the errors listed in figure 5.1.

CMS considers some codes (such as V57.2X, V57.3, V57.89, and V57.9) unacceptable for use as a principal diagnosis unless they carry a secondary diagnosis code describing the origin of the impairment. If the provider submits a claim that reports one of these codes as principal diagnosis without the necessary secondary diagnosis, the claim will be returned requesting a secondary diagnosis code. See figure 5.2 for examples.

When an invalid discharge status is reported, the patient is presumed (for the purpose of performing the nonspecific principal diagnosis check) to have been discharged alive.

How the Rules Relate to Legislation to Combat Fraud and Abuse

As part of the ongoing fraud and abuse prevention legislation, penalties can be assessed against anyone who engages in a "pattern of presenting a claim for an item or service based on a code the person knows or should know will result in greater payment than appropriate" (HHS 2000). The phrase "knows or should know" is interpreted as if the guideline was published in ICD-9-CM Official Guidelines for Coding and Reporting, or published and disseminated by the federal government or fiscal intermediary (FI)/Medicare Administrative Contractor (MAC) through provider bulletins or memoranda. Coders must have access to these publications on a regular basis in order to remain current on all regulations and guidelines as published. Moreover, coding staff should have regular meetings to share the content of these publications to ensure that all coders are following the same rules, as these rules may change frequently.

Key Resources for the Clinical Coding Specialist

Each hospital should have at least a minimal set of references for coders, such as those listed in annotated bibliography (pp. 219–220). The library should include a subscription to *Coding Clinic*, medical disease references, laboratory references, a medical dictionary, and drug references. If the facility utilizes an encoder tool, most of these references are included. As rules change, coders are advised to check frequently for updated guidance and information.

Figure 5.1.   Examples of errors that MCEs are designed to detect

- *Invalid diagnosis or procedure codes:* Each diagnosis or procedure code is checked against a listing of codes included in ICD-9-CM volume 1 (Diseases) and volume 3 (Procedures) to ensure its validity.

- *Invalid fourth or fifth digit:* Any diagnosis (including the admitting diagnosis) or procedure requiring a fourth or fifth digit that is either missing or not valid for the code in question.

- *E code as principal diagnosis:* An E code describes the circumstance that caused an injury, not the nature of the injury. Therefore, an E code should not be used as a principal diagnosis.

- *Duplicate diagnosis:* The MCE detects when the principal diagnosis is duplicated as a secondary diagnosis. For example, a coder assigns 800.12 twice because a patient has a closed frontal bone fracture with cerebral laceration and a closed parietal bone fracture with cerebral laceration and contusion. Because both fractures are assigned the same number, only one code is required. This edit was included because the duplicate code may be considered a significant complication or comorbidity that may result in assignment to an inappropriate DRG.

- *Age conflicts:* Age conflicts are inconsistencies between a patient's age and any diagnosis on the patient's claim. For example, code 779.0, Convulsions in newborn, should not appear on the record of an elderly patient. Four age categories are evaluated:

  —Diagnoses intended only for newborns and neonates with an age of 0, such as 775.1, Neonatal diabetes mellitus

  —Diagnoses considered reasonable only for children between 0 and 17 years, such as 331.81, Reye's syndrome

  —Maternity diagnoses that are usually valid only for patients between the ages of 12 and 55 years, such as 646.60, Infections of genitourinary tract in pregnancy

  —Diagnostic codes considered valid only for patients over the age of 14 years, such as 600.00 Hypertrophy (benign) of the prostate without urinary obstruction and other lower urinary tract symptoms

- *Sex conflicts:* Sex conflicts are inconsistencies between a diagnosis or procedure on the claim and the patient's sex. For example, a male patient is reported with uterine cancer or an oophorectomy. In both instances, the codes conflict with the stated sex. Therefore, the patient's diagnosis, procedure, or sex is presumed to be incorrect.

- *Manifestation code as a principal diagnosis:* These codes describe the manifestation of an underlying disease, not the disease itself. Therefore, they cannot be used as the principal diagnosis. Claims with these diagnoses will be returned to the healthcare facility. In volume 1 of the ICD-9-CM codebook, these codes have been italicized. A partial listing of the most common etiology codes that should be listed appropriately before a given italicized code also is provided. Because there are so many underlying causes for a given manifestation code, other etiological codes also may be used.

- *Nonspecific principal diagnoses:* Although unspecified diagnosis codes (particularly those designated as "not otherwise specified") are valid ICD-9-CM codes, a more precise code should be used, when possible, for the principal diagnosis. However, unspecified codes may be necessary on the claims of deceased patients because a patient who died may not have received a complete diagnostic workup. The Medicare contractor reviews bills submitted by providers for this exception type and determine whether provider education is necessary. Some intermediaries reject such claims for payment; others release them and then review them on a postpayment basis. To help educate physicians on this issue, the MCE generates a report for nonspecific principal diagnosis claims. The code editor program considers these valid ICD-9-CM codes insufficient for making Medicare coverage determinations.

- *Questionable admission:* The code edit detects diagnoses that do not usually provide sufficient justification for admission to an acute care hospital. Quality improvement organizations (QIOs), which are responsible for ensuring that appropriate care is rendered to Medicare beneficiaries in the appropriate setting, review questionable admission cases on a postpayment basis. Examples of a diagnosis that might precipitate a questionable admission flag would be benign hypertension or uncomplicated diabetes.

- *Unacceptable principal diagnoses:* Certain codes describe a circumstance that influences an individual's overall health status but has no specific bearing on a current illness or injury. For example, code V16.6, Family History of Leukemia, does not specifically explain why a patient was admitted. CMS considers such codes "unacceptable" for use as a principal diagnosis. If a provider files a claim using an "unacceptable principal diagnosis" code, that claim is returned with a request for a principal diagnosis describing the illness or injury. Some unacceptable principal diagnoses, such as benign hypertension, also are included on the questionable admission list.

Figure 5.2.   Codes that CMS considers unacceptable for principal diagnosis unless they carry a secondary diagnosis code

- *Nonspecific operating room procedures:* These procedures include a set of operating room (OR) procedure codes, particularly those described as "not otherwise specified." Although these codes are valid according to the ICD-9-CM coding scheme, more precise codes should be used. For example, rather than use 79.20, Open reduction of fracture without internal fixation, unspecified site, a code specifying the site should be used.

- *Noncovered operating room procedures:* The Medicare program does not provide payment for certain procedures. When one of these procedure codes is reported, the FI that pays for Medicare will return the bill as a no pay and request either a correction in the procedure code or a bill that identifies the covered and noncovered procedures. Included in the noncovered OR procedures are those procedures that Medicare has determined are not proven to be efficacious. Code 37.35, Partial ventriculectomy (ventricular reduction surgery), performed for treatment of end-stage heart failure due to cardiomyopathy, is an example of a noncovered OR procedure, as is code 37.52, Implantation of total replacement heart system (artificial heart).

- *Open-biopsy check:* Biopsies can be performed as open, percutaneous, or endoscopic procedures. The DRG definitions assign patients to different DRGs depending on whether the biopsy was open. In general, open biopsies are performed infrequently for most organ systems. There are specific ICD-9-CM codes for open and closed biopsies. Because the distinction made by the different biopsy codes is not applied uniformly, the MCE identifies all biopsies that are coded as open. When an open biopsy appears as either the principal or the secondary procedure, the FI may contact the hospital prior to payment to verify the procedure and obtain an operative report. If the operative report substantiates an open biopsy, the claim is processed. If the operative report reveals that the biopsy was performed percutaneously, by punch, or scope, the procedure code on the bill is changed to the corresponding closed-biopsy code before processing.

- *Medicare secondary payer alert:* The code editor will help contractors identify patients who may be covered under automobile insurance, workers' compensation, or other liability insurance. In such instances, Medicare should be the secondary payer. Claims with trauma codes are checked to determine which payer has primary responsibility for the claim.

- *Invalid age:* A patient's age is usually necessary for DRG determination. If the age reported is not between 0 and 124 years, the MCE will assume the age is in error.

- *Invalid sex:* A patient's sex is sometimes necessary for appropriate DRG determination. The sex code reported must be either 1 (male) or 2 (female).

- *Invalid patient status (discharge disposition):* A patient's discharge status is necessary for appropriate DRG determination. Patient status must be coded according to UB-04 definitions and conventions, for example:

  01   Discharged to home or self-care (routine discharge)

  02   Discharged/transferred to another short-term general hospital for inpatient care

  03   Discharged/transferred to Medicare-certified skilled nursing facility (SNF) (For hospitals with an approved swing bed arrangement, use code 61, Swing bed. For reporting discharges/transfers to a noncertified SNF, use code 04-ICF.)

  04   Discharged/transferred to an intermediate care facility (ICF)

  05   Discharged/transferred to another type of institution (including distinct parts)

  06   Discharged/transferred to home under care of organized home health service organization

  07   Left against medical advice or discontinued care

  08   Discharged/transferred to home under care of home IV drug therapy provider

  09   Admitted as an inpatient to this hospital

  10–19 Discharge to be defined at state level, if necessary

  20   Expired (or did not recover—Christian Science patient)

(Continued on next page)

Figure 5.2.   (Continued)

30	Still patient
40	Expired at home (hospice claims only)
41	Expired in a medical facility, such as a hospital, SNF, ICF, or freestanding hospice (hospice claims only)
42	Expired—place unknown (hospice claims only)
43	Discharged/transferred to a federal hospital (effective 10/1/03)
50	Hospice—home
51	Hospice—medical facility
61	Discharged/transferred within this institution to a hospital-based Medicare-approved swing bed
62	Discharged/transferred to an inpatient rehabilitation facility (IRF), including rehabilitation-distinct parts of a hospital
63	Discharged/transferred to a Medicare-certified long-term care hospital (LTCH)
64	Discharged/transferred to a nursing facility certified under Medicaid, but not certified under Medicare
71	Discharged/transferred/referred to another institution for outpatient services as specified by the discharge plan of care
72	Discharged/transferred/referred to this institution for outpatient services as specified by the discharge plan of care

Summary

Because coding today is tied directly to reimbursement of the facility, coders must understand many rules, regulations, and laws. This knowledge must be combined with clinical knowledge and skill to interpret clinical documentation and apply coding rules and guidelines to make accurate code assignment. Moreover, facilities must provide the training and resources necessary to ensure that coders maintain competency and stay abreast of changes that affect appropriate coding and billing.

Chapter 6

Coding and DRG Assignment

All coders must be ready to make decisions. The ICD-9-CM codebook contains about 13,000 diagnostic terms, but the Alphabetic Index recognizes more than 120,000 such terms. Additionally, physicians use thousands of terms not included in the Alphabetic Index and the coder must decide how to translate them into numerical designations. Although some coding discrepancies will inevitably occur, errors can be kept to a minimum if coders adhere to the following recommendations from the American Health Information Management Association (AHIMA) (AHIMA 2003):

- Use the complete health record as the coding source document.

- Employ qualified coding professionals with ongoing education and training in coding systems.

- Develop written coding policies that conform to the Uniform Hospital Discharge Data Set (UHDDS) definitions and the Cooperating Parties' official coding guidelines.

- Establish quality control procedures to monitor the consistency and completeness of code assignment.

Finally, persons who assign and report codes should always remember that it is unethical to manipulate codes to maximize reimbursement in ways that do not conform to the UHDDS definitions or guidelines.

The ability to review a health record and accurately assign the appropriate ICD-9-CM codes is a skill developed over an extended period of time. To become an expert at coding, one must have an understanding of disease processes and treatment. For accuracy and compliance in coding, the coder must rely on the documentation provided by physicians involved with the care of the patient, including both the attending physician and any consultants he or she deems necessary to assist with patient care. This chapter discusses the basic parts of a health record, what the coder should look for in each part, and the steps in a record review that coders should follow to determine principal diagnosis.

Circumstances of Admission

The guidelines indicate that the circumstances of inpatient admission always govern the selection of principal diagnosis. The circumstances of the admission are determined by reviewing the documentation contained in the health record.

The health record entries made at the time of admission should be reviewed carefully to identify why the patient was admitted. For patients entering through the emergency department, the coder should identify the symptoms, findings, and/or diagnoses recorded in the emergency department record. Often the emergency department record will clearly identify the diagnosis necessitating admission. In other health records, however, the documentation may not be so clear and it may be necessary to review additional sources of information, such as:

- The admitting diagnosis listed on the face sheet

- The physician's conclusions recorded in the history and physical examination

- The patient's chief complaint as recorded on the nursing assessment, history, and physical examination

- The initial and subsequent progress notes

- Reports by consultants who saw the patient soon after admission

- The initial orders to identify the focus of treatment (Most hospitals require that the admission diagnosis be recorded as part of the admission order, although this diagnosis may be quite vague.)

Progress note documentation is especially relevant for patients admitted with symptoms or physical findings that require further study to identify underlying causes. In the progress notes, the physician records the results of studies being performed, assesses the patient's status, and draws the conclusion when all studies are performed.

Data recorded at or near the time of admission are more useful in identifying the circumstances of the admission than the discharge summary or final progress notes because these documents contain information related to the patient's condition at the time of discharge. Thus, the physician may focus on the most significant diagnosis in terms of implications for the patient's health, medical care, and use of the hospital. If death occurs, the physician may record the cause of death instead of identifying why the patient was admitted.

In most instances, it is possible to identify the principal diagnosis with a high degree of certainty after carefully reviewing health record documentation. However, there may be problems with ambiguous, incomplete, or conflicting documentation. In such instances, documentation deficiencies should be queried, according to facility policy, with the physician or the appropriate medical staff committee.

Identifying the Sections of the Health Record

Every health record is composed of five basic sections:

1. An initial database

2. Consultations

3. Diagnostic tests

4. Therapeutic procedures

5. Daily documentation

Initial Database

The initial database consists of the emergency department record (if applicable) and the patient's history and physical examination. This initial information will provide a key to the potential principal diagnosis.

History and Physical

The history and the physical examination need to be reviewed for two types of information. The first type of information can influence identification of the principal diagnosis and includes the following:

- The chief complaint
- The history of present illness
- Current medications
- Presenting physical signs and symptoms

The second type of information can influence the number and types of additional diagnoses, which are considered secondary diagnoses. This information may include identification of potential complications to the principal diagnosis. For example, a review of the patient's current medications may make it possible to identify stable conditions that are presently under treatment and that should be reported as secondary diagnoses, such as acute diastolic heart failure, acute exacerbation of chronic obstructive pulmonary disease (COPD), type I or type II diabetes, hypertension, or peptic ulcer disease. Any diagnosis identified in this review must be confirmed by physician documentation in the final diagnostic statement. If questions arise about whether a diagnosis should be reported, the physician should be consulted for confirmation.

Although not all-encompassing, the list in table 6.1 represents common medications associated with typical secondary diagnoses.

Consultations

If the attending physician requests consultations from specialists, their reports should be reviewed for support of the potential principal diagnosis, as well as significant secondary

Table 6.1.   Examples of common medications associated with secondary diagnoses

Diagnoses	Common Medications
Hypertension	Dyazide, Propranolol, Captopril
COPD	Theophylline, Aminophylline, Theo-Dur
Angina	Nitrostat, Nitro Paste, Nitro-Bid
CHF	Lasix, Digoxin, Lanoxin
Peptic ulcer disease	Zantac, Tagamet, Pepcid

Diabetes mellitus
   Type I
   Type II
	Novolin, NPH, Humulin
	Orinase, Dymelor, Diabinese, Glucotrol

diagnoses. In some hospitals, diagnoses that are identified and treated by consultants are added routinely to the final list of diagnoses. However, the attending physician retains control of the patient's care throughout the hospital visit and is responsible for reviewing the documentation provided by the consulting physician(s) and assessing its significance for the patient. Hospital coding guidelines should address this issue. The attending physician reviews the reports provided by the consulting physician and assesses and documents the significance of the findings.

When a patient is admitted for surgery, a medical consultation report for "surgery clearance" may be present. Frequently, this type of consultation identifies significant medical conditions for which the patient is undergoing treatment that may influence the surgical outcome or length of stay (LOS). Such conditions should be added to the diagnostic statement when documented by the attending physician. When a condition is identified, but not documented, a query process should be started.

Diagnostic Tests

This section of the health record may help justify a principal diagnosis or support the coding of a secondary diagnosis. For example, in the case of a patient with suspected sepsis, a positive blood culture present on admission or within several hours after admission will usually support sepsis as a principal diagnosis, particularly when the record identifies the focus of treatment as such. Negative or inconclusive blood cultures, however, do not preclude a diagnosis of sepsis in a patient with clinical evidence of the condition.

Repeated monitoring of laboratory values or abnormal values followed by a treatment order may suggest the presence of a significant secondary diagnosis that also may be a complication or comorbidity. For example, repeated tests for potassium levels followed by orders for a potassium supplement would suggest hypokalemia as a secondary diagnosis, if verified by the attending physician. However, coders should always be cautious in reviewing diagnostic tests. Even though a value may be abnormal, an additional diagnosis should not be added unless the related condition is treated or meets the criteria for inclusion as a secondary diagnosis. In unclear cases, the coder is obligated to consult the attending physician. The *ICD-9-CM Official Guidelines for Coding and Reporting* (Section III, B) explain:

> Abnormal findings (laboratory, x-ray, pathologic, and other diagnostic results) are not coded and reported unless the physician indicates their clinical significance. If the findings are outside the normal range and the attending physician has ordered other tests to evaluate the condition or prescribed treatment, it is appropriate to ask the physician whether the abnormal finding should be added.

Any cultures of body fluids also should be reviewed because they may assist in identifying bacterial infections that would influence the patient's treatment. When these diagnostic tests indicate that a secondary condition may be present, the coder should review the progress notes for the attending or consulting physician's comments for documentation of possible additional diagnoses. (Refer to the discussion of progress in the section below on daily documentation.)

Therapeutic Procedures

As the treatment pattern begins to emerge, therapeutic procedures may be used to correct particular problems. These procedures may or may not influence MS-DRG assignment. For example, a case of angina with a cardiac catheterization and subsequent coronary artery bypass graft (CABG) procedure will be assigned to a different DRG than a case of angina with only a cardiac catheterization.

Therapeutic procedures may be performed in an operating room or at the patient's bedside and still have an impact on the DRG assignment. For example, different DRGs would be assigned for the following two patients:

Example: Patient A is admitted with decubitus ulcers. The ulcers are conservatively treated with IV antibiotics, repeat scrubbing, and topical medications.

Patient B is admitted with the same diagnosis, but the ulcers are débrided with a scalpel at the bedside.

Procedures such as the sharp débridement of skin ulcers using scalpel to "bleeding" tissue at the patient's bedside require close review of the progress notes because that may be the only method of identifying that the procedure was performed. Of course, these procedures also may be performed in the operating room.

Daily Documentation

One of the most important sections of the health record, daily documentation, usually includes the physician and allied health progress notes, physician orders, flow sheets for critical care, ventilator support, and ancillary records.

The physician orders will help identify the focus of treatment and support selection of the principal diagnosis. Here, the coordination of care can be located. It is important to coordinate the review of diagnostic tests and consultations to appropriately identify not only the principal diagnosis, but also significant secondary conditions. This is the place to find the patient's current medications for "stable" types of chronic problems that might still affect patient management in the current episode of care.

The progress notes provided by the physician and allied health team will document the patient's response to treatments. Moreover, they serve as backup documentation for various diagnostic and therapeutic procedures until a dictated report is provided. The coder should review the notes carefully to determine whether LOS was affected by secondary diagnoses or whether a complication developed postoperatively. For example, it may be possible to identify a postoperative complication of urinary retention by noting whether the patient had to be recatheterized or whether he or she was given a dose of diuretics to restart the passage of urine after surgery. Complication must be documented by the physician, or the coder may query for the cause and effect relationship.

Reviewing the Health Record

Each section of the health record serves a separate purpose. When reviewed correctly by the clinical coding professional, the sections taken together will support or justify the principal diagnosis and any secondary conditions that might affect reimbursement. It is important to remember that, in order to be coded, these conditions must be appropriately documented by the physician. When the documentation is incomplete, ambiguous, or conflicting, a physician query is in order. See appendix C (p. 173) for a sample physician query form.

A suggested sequence of review follows. The coder should:

1. Determine if an *emergency department record* is attached and, if so, review physician documentation and any comments from the ambulance report for pertinent information.

2. Review the *admission orders* to confirm any suspected principal diagnosis and/or to support the admitting diagnosis.

3. Read the *history and physical examination* to determine admitting diagnoses that may be categorized as the principal diagnosis and to identify potentially codeable secondary diagnoses.

4. Read the *consultation reports* from specialists that may further support or refute the potential principal diagnosis and/or potentially codeable secondary diagnoses.

5. Read all *progress notes* and develop a sense of the focus of treatment, progression of signs, and symptoms to diagnoses.

6. Verify any potential secondary diagnoses with *laboratory, radiology,* or *other ancillary tests, progress notes,* and *physician orders* and identify need to query.

7. Read the *operative reports, pathology reports, discharge summary* and/or *special procedures or reports* to confirm primary and secondary diagnoses and procedures and identify need to query.

8. Identify the *principal diagnosis* and, when necessary, confirm appropriateness with the attending physician.

9. Develop a *list of secondary diagnoses* to be reported and, when needed, verify with the attending physician to ensure accuracy.

10. *Code all relevant diagnoses* following ethical coding standards and the UHDDS official guidelines.

Querying the Physician

As stated throughout this chapter, there are times when documentation is incomplete or insufficient to support the diagnoses found in the chart. It is for this reason that facilities should establish a physician query policy. Coders and physicians need to be familiar with the policy and procedures to ensure that this process works as smoothly as possible. The most common way of querying the physician is through the use of a query form.

Query Forms

Query forms should be developed and used with care and should only be used as tools to facilitate communication between coder and physician. The facility should develop a standardized form with input from both coders and physicians. Usually, the query form is not considered part of the official legal medical record. AHIMA recommends that facilities choosing to incorporate the form into their medical record should do so only under guidance from legal counsel and the compliance department in order to avoid problems such as "potential use as evidence of poor documentation in an audit, investigation or malpractice suit" (Prophet 2001).

The coder should keep to factual/clinical information (clinical indicators) and should not "lead" the physician toward a particular answer. Questions asked should remain open ended to allow the physician to improve documentation. The physician should be guided toward clarifying any discrepancies in the body of the documentation, rather than just replying on the query form. This can be accomplished through use of an addendum to the discharge summary or progress notes.

According to Prophet (2001):

The goal of the query process should be to improve physician documentation and coding professionals' understanding of the unique clinical situation, not to improve reimbursement. Each facility should establish a policy and procedure for obtaining physician clarification of documentation that affects code assignment. The process of querying physicians must be a patient-specific process, not a general process.

See appendix C (pp. 165–173) for AHIMA's practice brief on Developing a Physician Query Process (2001).

The facility should ensure that its query policy follows Medicare, Joint Commission, and facility documentation guidelines, as well as official coding guidelines. Coders should be encouraged to query the physician when the documentation is unclear or ambiguous; however, coders should not use the process to diagnose or question the physician's medical judgment.

Clinical Documentation Improvement Program (CDIP)

Over the years, many facilities have struggled over when to begin the coding process. Traditionally, the chart is coded after the patient's encounter or episode of care is complete. If documentation is clear and complete, then the coder should have all the information needed to accurately assign codes to the patient's diagnoses and procedures. However, if information is missing or ambiguous, obtaining answers to coding queries is difficult and time-consuming once the patient has been discharged and the clinician has moved on to treating other patients. As Medicare and other payers look to improve patient care and provide more accurate payment based on the patient's documented severity of illness, organizations are retooling their coding process.

One such alternative to the retrospective querying process is commonly known as a Clinical Documentation Improvement Program (CDIP). Coders work together with nursing staff and/or case managers to help ensure that clinical documentation is sufficient to support the patient's medical care. This process is designed to enhance patient care through better documentation. It also allows for a smoother coding process because any documentation issues are identified in real time instead of days or weeks after the patient has been treated.

Clinical documentation specialists (CDS) are coding professionals and nurses who work on the patient floors or alongside the physicians in the clinic setting. Although some facilities may choose nursing staff for this position, coding professionals also are excellent candidates. It is imperative that the CDS has a mixture of coding and clinical knowledge and possesses the communication skills necessary to query physicians and other clinicians when questions arise regarding the medical documentation. In the physician clinic setting, the CDS may also review inpatient chart documentation to facilitate correct coding for the physician's professional services. This task also requires a strong working relationship between the hospital and physician practice (Scott 2008).

Present on Admission

Portions of this section are adapted from *Present on Admission* (Garrett 2007).

With the implementation of the UB-04 billing form in 2007, an additional field was added to allow for indication of whether each diagnosis was "present on admission" (POA).

Reasons for the addition of the POA indicator are included in the MEDPAC Report to the Congress (2005, 191):

> Currently, a diagnosis recorded on the discharge summary that may have been present on admission cannot be distinguished from one that developed during the hospital stay. This additional information would significantly enhance the ability to identify which complications are avoidable. It would improve risk-adjustment of mortality and complications measures. Several quality organizations have supported this concept, and it should not significantly increase hospital burden.

The POA indicator is required to be addressed on all short-term inpatient admission claims. It is designed to identify conditions that are diagnosed prior to admission and conditions diagnosed during admission that were clearly present but not diagnosed until after admission occurred. Any condition that was present at the time the order for inpatient admission occurs, including conditions that develop during an outpatient encounter, such as emergency department, observation, or outpatient surgery, are considered as present on admission.

The POA indicator is assigned to the principal and secondary diagnoses and the external cause of injury codes except where exempt from reporting. Appendix I was added to the Official Coding Guidelines to define and explain proper usage of the POA indicator (NCHS 2007, 92–105). According to these guidelines, POA is *not* intended to replace any coding guidelines in the main body of ICD-9-CM *Official Guidelines for Coding and Reporting* and is *not* to provide guidance on when a condition should be coded.

Short-term acute care hospitals began reporting the POA on each diagnosis code on October 1, 2007, by using one of four indicators.

1. Y = Yes, the condition was present on admission

2. N = No, the condition was not present on admission

3. W = Clinically undetermined (the provider is unable to clinically determine if the condition was present on admission)

4. U = Unknown. This indicator shows that the chart documentation is insufficient to determine whether or not the condition was present on admission. The U indicator should not be used much as it should serve to prompt the coder to query the physician for additional information.

To further facilities down the path of "pay for performance" (P4P), CMS was required by law to select at least two conditions that will be excluded from the payment calculations if they are acquired during the hospitalization. This will result in a decrease in reimbursement to hospitals if the condition is a complication or comorbidity (CC) or major complication or comorbidity (MCC) and occurred after the patient was admitted to the hospital.

The following information from the August 1, 2007, Final Changes to the Hospital Inpatient Prospective Payment System, Final Rule, summarizes the next steps (as quoted in Garrett 2008, 5):

> Per Section 5001 (c) of Public law 109-171 requires the Secretary to select, by October 1, 2007, at least two conditions that are (a) high cost or high volume or both, (b) result in the assignment of a case to a DRG that has a higher payment when present as a secondary diagnosis, and (c) could reasonably have been prevented through application of evidence-based guidelines. For discharges occurring on or after October 1, 2008, hospitals will not receive additional payment

for cases in which the selected conditions were not present on admission. That is, the case will be paid as though the secondary diagnosis was not present. Section 5001(c) provides that we can revise the list of conditions. Section 5001(c) also requires hospitals to submit the secondary diagnoses that are present at admission when reporting payment information for discharges on or after October 1, 2007.

The following criteria were applied to select the final list of conditions:

1. **Coding:** Easily identified by unique ICD-9-CM codes

2. **Burden:** High cost, high volume, or both

3. **Prevention guidelines:** Could reasonably have been prevented through the application of evidence-based guidelines

4. **CC/MCC:** Assignment of a case to a DRG that has a higher payment when the code is present as a CC or MCC.

5. **Considerations:** How condition meets statutory criteria in light of potential difficulties that CMS would face if the condition were selected

In the Final Rule, CMS lists the hospital-acquired conditions that it will use to meet the Deficit Reduction Act (DRA) requirements. How each condition met the above criteria, as well as information about those that did not, is also discussed in detail in the final rule. Beginning in FY 2009 (Oct. 1, 2008), cases with the following conditions will not be paid at a higher rate unless the conditions were present on admission:

- Catheter-associated urinary tract infection

- Pressure ulcers

- Object left in body during surgery

- Air embolism

- Delivery of ABO-incompatible blood products

- Vascular catheter-associated infections

- Mediastinitis after CABG surgery

- Falls and fractures, dislocations, intracranial and crushing injury, and burns

Although these CMS requirements have shifted the focus of attention to assigning these indicators to Medicare claims, it is important to note that the POA requirement is described in the Official Coding Guidelines, as stated above. POA is not just to be addressed on Medicare patients only. The POA indicator should be added to all claims for all diagnoses that meet the criteria as established in the Official Coding Guidelines.

Other Guidelines for Reporting Diagnoses

When patients have multiple diagnoses, it is sometimes difficult for the coding professional to find clear evidence of the ONE that best meets the definition of principal diagnosis. When questions arise, the Official Coding Guidelines provide examples and instructions to assist in the appropriate selection of principal diagnosis. There are also specific instructions found to assist the coding professional in assignment of secondary codes.

Symptoms, Signs, and Ill-Defined Conditions

Manifestations are characteristic signs or symptoms of an illness. Signs and symptoms that pertain to a given diagnosis and primarily affect a specific body system are assigned to categories in chapters 1 through 15 of the Tabular List in the ICD-9-CM codebook.

Examples: 276.2 Acidosis
578.0 Hematemesis

ICD-9-CM chapter 16 (categories 780–799) includes symptoms and signs that point to two or more diseases or two or more systems of the body, abnormal results of laboratory or other investigative procedures, and ill-defined conditions in which no diagnosis classifiable elsewhere is recorded. These codes should not be used to identify a principal diagnosis when a related definitive diagnosis is available.

A sign or symptom code may be used instead of a diagnosis code and may possibly constitute the principal diagnosis in the following instances:

- No more specific diagnosis can be made at the time of discharge or outpatient encounter.

- The transient nature of the signs and symptoms makes it impossible to identify the cause.

- The patient does not return or expires before evaluation permits complete workup.

- The patient is referred elsewhere before a diagnosis is made.

- A more precise diagnosis is unavailable.

- The adverse reaction a patient experiences to a drug is a symptom code.

- The symptom or sign is a sequela related to a late effect of an illness or injury.

When the cause of a symptom or sign is stated in the diagnosis, the coder should report the code identifying the cause. An additional code may be assigned to further identify the symptom or sign when it represents an important problem in medical care on which data may need to be tracked.

Example: Brain metastasis, 198.3
Coma, 780.01

Comatose patients require extra care, so this symptom is reported in addition to the cause.

Example: Leukocytosis, nausea, and vomiting due to acute appendicitis

Only the acute appendicitis would be coded (540.9) because the symptoms specified are signs and symptoms of appendicitis. There is no need to maintain data on these signs and symptoms unless they persist following surgery.

In some circumstances, the symptom may be the sole reason for admission. When a patient is admitted for the purpose of treating the symptom, and there is no treatment or further evaluation of the underlying disease, the symptom can be designated as the principal diagnosis. Often the symptom represents an acute problem caused by a long-standing chronic condition that does not justify hospital admission. In all cases, sequencing of the diagnoses depends on the circumstances of the current admission or encounter.

Example: Back pain management due to chronic lumbosacral strain

Because the treatment is specifically for back pain, it would be coded as the principal diagnosis, even though the pain is a symptom of a chronic condition.

Reporting of Other (Additional) Diagnoses

A joint effort between the attending physician and coding professional is essential to achieve complete and accurate documentation, code assignment, and diagnosis and procedure reporting. To assist both the physician and coder, the Cooperating Parties developed and approved specific guidelines for identifying which diagnoses to report in addition to the principal diagnosis. Hospitals may record other diagnoses, as needed, for internal data use.

UHDDS definitions are used by short-term acute care hospitals to report inpatient data elements in a standardized manner. These data elements and their definitions can be found in the July 31, 1985, *Federal Register* (HHS 1985).

UHDDS item #ll-b defines "other diagnoses" as (HHS 1985):

All conditions that coexist at the time of admission, that develop subsequently, or that affect the treatment received and/or the length of stay. Diagnoses that relate to an earlier episode which have no bearing on the current hospital stay are to be excluded.

General Rule

For reporting purposes, the definition of "other diagnoses" is interpreted as additional conditions that affect patient care by requiring any of the following:

- Evaluation

- Therapeutic treatment or diagnostic procedures

- Extended LOS

- Increased nursing care, increased monitoring, or both

The following guidelines are to be applied in designating other diagnoses when neither the Alphabetic Index nor the Tabular List in the ICD-9-CM codebook provides direction.

Previous Conditions

Ordinarily, diagnoses the physician has included in the final diagnostic statement (such as those appearing in the discharge summary or the face sheet) should be reported, but some physicians include historical information or status post procedures performed on a previous admission that have no bearing on the current stay. Such conditions are not to be reported. However, history codes (V10–V19) may be used as secondary codes when the historical condition or family history has an impact on current care or influences treatment (ICD-9-CM Official Guidelines for Coding and Reporting, Section III, A).

Diagnoses Not Listed in the Final Diagnostic Statement

When the physician has documented what appears to be a current diagnosis in the body of the record but has not included it in the final diagnostic statement, the coding professional should ask the physician to add the current diagnosis. However, according to guidance found in *Coding Clinic*, coders are allowed to code diagnoses from the body of the record (AHA 2000, 17):

> As long as documentation is clear and consistent, the coder may assign codes if they meet the definition of other diagnoses. If the coder is uncertain whether it is a valid diagnosis because the documentation is incomplete, vague, or contradictory, then the coder should query the physician to determine if the diagnosis should be a part of the final diagnostic statement.

Conditions That Are an Integral Part of a Disease Process

Conditions that are an integral part of a disease process should not be assigned as additional codes.

Conditions That Are Not an Integral Part of a Disease Process

Additional conditions that may not be associated routinely with a disease process should be coded when present. For example, when a patient is admitted with chest pain, but it is found after study that the patient had referred chest pain due to gastroesophageal reflux disease (GERD), the chest pain would be coded separately to justify the tests performed to evaluate the cause of this symptom, such as EKGs and Troponin levels.

Abnormal Findings

Abnormal findings (laboratory, x-ray, pathologic, and other diagnostic results) are not assigned or reported unless the physician indicates their clinical significance. If the findings are outside the normal range and the attending physician has ordered other tests to evaluate the condition or prescribed treatment, it is appropriate for the coder to ask the physician whether the diagnosis should be added.

Angina

When a patient is admitted for another reason but is taking medication for angina, the angina is reportable as an additional diagnosis. It is considered to be under treatment even though the condition is stable and the patient has no episodes during the current stay. The condition is reportable if the physician includes angina in the diagnostic statement. The physician may state that the condition is compensated or stable.

Congestive Heart Failure

When a patient with a history of congestive heart failure (CHF) is admitted for another reason and is currently taking medication for CHF (such as Digoxin and Lasix with a potassium supplement), the CHF should be reported. The patient would continue on the medications during the current stay even if no signs of cardiac decompensation are present. The physician may describe this type of CHF as compensated, stable, or history of CHF. It is still reportable as an additional diagnosis. The coding professional should also review the medical documentation to determine if the heart failure is specified as acute versus chronic and diastolic, systolic, or both diastolic and systolic. This specificity will impact the selection of the correct coding assignment and the MS-DRG assignment impacting reimbursement since CHF no longer counts as a CC.

Frequently Overlooked Diagnoses

Coders should examine the entire health record carefully for conditions and statements that may indicate additional diagnoses. Remember that in order to code these conditions, they need to be documented by the physician or the potential diagnosis should be queried. The following list is an example of clues for diagnoses that are frequently overlooked in reporting:

- Anemia
    - —Faintness, dizziness, pallor, fatigue, thirst, sweating, blood loss (for instance, ulcer, trauma, hematemesis, or melena)
    - —Low hemoglobin or hematocrit
    - —Administration of iron or blood components
- Cardiac arrhythmias (especially in patients with acute myocardial infarctions)
    - —Palpitations, near syncope, pallor, nausea, weakness, lightheadedness, fatigue
    - —EKG findings confirmed by a physician as clinically significant
    - —Cardioversion, Digitalis, Verapamil therapy, beta- or calcium blockers, pacemaker insertion
- Dehydration (especially in patients with gastroenteritis or those who are eating poorly)
    - —History of diarrhea or vomiting, dry mucous membranes, poor skin turgor, weakness
    - —Elevated BUN, electrolyte imbalance
    - —Force fluids, IV rehydration (for instance, >125 cc/hr)
- Urinary tract infection (especially in postoperative patients and those admitted from nursing homes)
    - —Dysuria, urinary urgency and frequency, flank pain or tenderness, possible fever, chills, and general malaise
    - —WBCs, RBCs, and bacteria on urinalysis, urine culture positive for organism causing infection (colony count greater than 100,000)
    - —Antibiotic therapy, force fluids
- Heart failure (especially in patients with respiratory disease or other cardiac conditions)
    - —Dyspnea, orthopnea, peripheral edema, rales
    - —Positive chest x-ray (pulmonary venous congestion)
    - —Lasix, Digoxin, low-salt diet, oxygen administration

- Gastrointestinal bleeding (especially in patients with severe gastritis or those taking large quantities of anti-inflammatory drugs)

  —Fatigue, pallor, dizziness, hematemesis, or melena

  —Low hemoglobin/hematocrit, stool positive for occult blood, endoscopy confirmation, upper and lower GI series

  —Blood replacement, NG tube, special diet, antacid prescribed

- Chronic obstructive pulmonary disease

  —Shortness of breath on exertion, dyspnea, chronic intermittent cough or wheezing

  —Positive chest x-ray, increased residual volume and decreased vital capacity on pulmonary function tests, abnormal blood gases, low Theophylline levels

  —Treatment focuses on relieving symptoms and preventing exacerbations

  —Chest physiotherapy, bronchodilator, oxygen therapy, corticosteroids

  —Chronic condition versus an (acute) exacerbation of the COPD

- Malnutrition (especially in patients admitted from nursing homes)

  —Low weight, lethargy

  —Poor appetite

  —Insertion of feeding tube, total parenteral nutrition, nutritional supplements

- Status or disabilities

  —Blindness, deafness, absence of limb, presence of colostomy requiring extra nursing time, pacemaker status, aortocoronary bypass status, transplant status (may require extra testing or increase the risk associated with other diseases and procedures)

Frequently Overlooked Procedures

Following is a list of tips for identifying procedures that are frequently overlooked by physicians and coders:

- *Excisional débridement:* The coder should look for decubitus ulcers, diabetic foot ulcers, and/or cellulitis. Nursing and physical therapy notes also should be reviewed for documentation. Bedside procedures, such as excisional débridement, are frequently documented in the nursing notes. Moreover, physicians may perform this procedure during physical therapy. When this is the case, physical therapy notes should be reviewed to verify that the physician visited the patient during a session in the whirlpool and performed the débridement.

- *Adhesiolysis:* The coder should look for abdominal surgery on a patient with a history of previous abdominal procedures, hernia procedures on patients with a previous hernia procedure or a previous lower abdominal procedure, cholecystectomy procedures where the patient has a history of prior appendectomy, and/or a previous history of peritonitis or internal bleeding and ulceration. *Coding Clinic* requires documentation that the adhesiolysis was required in order to access the organ or site of the procedure.

- *Common bile duct exploration with cholecystectomy:* The coder should review the procedure dictation to find documentation that states the surgeon needed to explore the common bile duct for stones. This may be performed with open-cholecystectomy procedures. An intraoperative cholangiogram is a diagnostic radiological procedure to assess the bile ducts. Dye is injected into the bile ducts to assess for the presence of stones or other abnormalities. This is not the same as a common bile duct exploration; a common duct exploration can be performed open, transendoscopically via ERCP with endoscopic sphincterotomy, or laparoscopically, but it always requires an incision into the common bile duct and manipulation of the common bile duct to some extent.

- *Bone graft harvesting:* For certain spinal fusions or bone procedures for fracture non-unions, it may be necessary to harvest bone from one anatomical site for use in another (77.70–77.79). Frequently, the bone (or bone marrow) is harvested from the iliac crest. The bone graft harvesting is included with some ICD-9-CM codes, such as limb-lengthening procedures (78.30–78.39), but not with others. The coder must review the codebook carefully prior to assigning an additional code.

- *Repair of inadvertent lacerations:* The coder should review operative notes carefully to identify the repair of accidental lacerations. If the surgeon must repair the inadvertent tear, the additional code for the suture of the site of the tear should be added.

- *Pacemaker insertions:* The coder should review progress notes and emergency department notes for insertions of pacemakers. Insertion of both the device and the lead or leads is coded.

- *Mechanical ventilation:* The coder should review progress notes and emergency department notes for the beginning time of mechanical ventilation. Ventilator flow sheets usually accompany the health record of a patient on mechanical ventilation. In some facilities, coding professionals are responsible for calculating total hours of mechanical ventilation based on documentation in the patient's record. Great care should be taken to follow ICD-9-CM instructions for counting both start time and stop time of mechanical ventilation.

- *Biopsies:* During the course of a major procedure, the surgeon may elect to take an unplanned biopsy of other structures. The coder should review the operative note carefully to identify the additional procedure.

Applying the Guidelines

The following case examples are designed to increase the understanding of, and ability to select, appropriate UHDDS principal and secondary diagnoses. The correct answers can be found at the end of the chapter.

Case 6.1

Patient A was admitted with shortness of breath and chest pain. He has a history of adenocarcinoma of the colon five years ago. At that time, he had a colonoscopy and biopsy with removal of malignant lesion, with no disease found in the resected colon. A chest x-ray revealed large pleural effusion. A thoracentesis was performed to remove a large amount of fluid, after which the patient's breathing and chest pain improved. Cytology revealed metastatic adenocarcinoma of the pleura. An oncology consultant examined the patient and felt that he was a candidate for chemotherapy. Initial treatment of 5FU, Methotrexate, and Cytoxan was given. The patient was discharged with a diagnosis of pleural effusion due to metastatic adenocarcinoma of the pleura.

Answer:

Principal Diagnosis: _____

Secondary Diagnoses: _____

Case 6.2

Patient B, an elderly female, was admitted from a nursing home with a history of poor appetite and marked weakness with lethargy for two days prior to admission. There was no history of diarrhea or vomiting. Mucous membranes were very dry and skin turgor was poor. The patient had no shortness of breath, chills, or fever. The nursing home BUN level was 65. IV therapy was started for hydration and nutrition. With hydration, the BUN decreased to 30. The patient became more alert and responsive to stimuli, and began eating. She was discharged to the nursing home clinically stable with diagnoses of dehydration, mild malnutrition causing weakness, and elevated BUN.

Answer:

Principal Diagnosis: _____

Secondary Diagnoses: _____

Case 6.3

Patient C is admitted with acute bronchopneumonia unresponsive to outpatient treatment. She has been on chemotherapy for previously resected breast carcinoma of the upper-inner quadrant. She has been on an eight-week regimen that started after her breast surgery. In addition, she has axillary and lung metastases. The pneumonia responded slowly to IV antibiotic therapy, but when her lungs cleared, the patient was discharged to resume antineoplastic therapy in one week.

Answer:

Principal Diagnosis: _____

Secondary Diagnoses: _____

Summary

The practice of clinical coding requires a unique blend of coding and clinical knowledge, skill, and judgment. Responsible coding professionals are able to read and interpret documentation in health records, clarify questions with physicians, and apply official coding guidelines accurately, consistently, and completely in assigning principal and secondary diagnoses, procedures, and other applicable codes. The expert coder is one who is aware of and respects the ethical issues in coding compliance.

Answers to Case Studies

Case 6.1

Principal Diagnosis: 197.2, Secondary malignant neoplasm of pleura. After study, the principal diagnosis of malignant pleural effusion was found to have been the cause of the shortness of breath and chest pain. These symptoms are not coded since a definitive diagnosis was found.

Secondary Diagnoses: V10.05, History of colon cancer. The history of colon cancer is used because there is documentation that the colon cancer was resected and without evidence of recurrence.

Case 6.2

Principal Diagnosis: 276.51, Dehydration. The principal diagnosis is dehydration because, after study, that is what was identified as the underlying cause of the weakness, lethargy, and increased BUN. Her appetite improved when she became more alert.

Secondary Diagnoses: 263.1, Malnutrition of mild degree should be reported as a secondary diagnosis.

Case 6.3

Principal Diagnosis: 485, Bronchopneumonia, organism unspecified. The principal diagnosis is acute broncho-pneumonia because therapy focused on this condition. The patient's stay was compli-cated by the metastatic carcinoma, as antineoplastic therapy exerts a suppressive action on the immune mechanisms, thus making the pneumonia more difficult to treat and extending the stay.

Secondary Diagnoses: 174.2, Malignant neoplasm of upper-inner quadrant.

197.0, Secondary malignant neoplasm of lung.

196.3, Secondary neoplasm of axillary lymph nodes.

The breast cancer is reported as current even though it has been surgically excised because it appears that the patient has been on chemotherapy since the surgery and, therefore, it is currently being treated. The metastatic sites of the lymph nodes and lung should be reported.

Part III

Processes Related to Coding and Reimbursement for Inpatient Services

Chapter 7

Data Quality Management

The need for clinical information in the form of coded data has been magnified dramatically since the beginning of the prospective payment system (PPS). Quality improvement organizations (QIOs), third-party administrators, fiscal intermediaries (FIs)/Medicare Administrative Contractors (MACs), employers, and commercial insurance groups rely on the data that health information management (HIM) professionals provide to make financial decisions and to validate quality of care. As reimbursement is directly tied to quality with the Value Based Purchasing and Pay for Performance Initiatives, the need for accurate and complete information has resulted in a close examination of the coding process within HIM services. This chapter focuses on the processes for evaluating, controlling, and monitoring the quality of healthcare data.

Coding and Data Quality Evaluation

Critical elements in the data quality evaluation process include:

- Coding practices and policies
- Staff qualifications
- Training
- Types of quality control programs

Coding managers play an important role in the data quality evaluation process. They are responsible for the following types of activities:

- Preparation of specific coding criteria
- Planning of coder educational sessions
- Evaluation and monitoring of educational action plans for individual coders
- Monitoring of ethical coding practices
- Evaluation and monitoring of coding quality
- Preparation of performance evaluations

Quality, as it applies to coded data, means that the performance of the coding function within an HIM department is accomplished at the highest level of accuracy and consistency possible for the coded data. Likewise, quality is expressed most appropriately in terms of the needs of the customers. That is, the definition of quality implies that optimal reimbursement is provided to the hospital, patients' illnesses and treatments are reported accurately, and payers can identify all the resources required to treat one of their beneficiaries.

As we face multiple transitions in the reimbursement system for government programs, an accurate database for planning is critical. The data that healthcare organizations provide today will have a profound impact on the future reimbursement they may expect. Large-scale data warehousing by organizations such as HealthGrades allows for greater data comparison and benchmarking. By describing the resources used for a patient completely and accurately, HIM professionals ensure that the database for reimbursement decisions is as detailed as possible.

AHIMA's Data Quality Management Model

Because the data in the health record must be of the highest quality to accomplish all the purposes required of it, in 1998 AHIMA developed a task force on the subject of data quality management. This group developed a data quality management model based on four domains and the basic characteristics that apply to them (Cassidy et al. 1998).

Quality Management Domains

Each of the four domains that form the framework of AHIMA's data quality management model represents a set of processes. These domains, with their associated processes, include:

- Data applications, or the purposes for which data are collected

- Data collection, or the processes by which data are collected

- Data warehousing, or the processes and systems by which data are archived or saved for future use

- Data analysis, or the processes by which data are translated into information that can be used for the designated application

Required Characteristics

The processes that result in high-quality data require certain characteristics, ranging from accuracy and accessibility to relevance and consistency. The characteristics that are applied to the four quality management domains in the AHIMA model are described in the following sections (adapted from Homan 2007, 36–41).

Accuracy

Data accuracy refers to the correctness of data. The data should represent what was intended or defined by their original source. For example, the patient's emergency contact information recorded in a paper record or a database should be the same as what the patient said it was. The results of laboratory testing for a particular patient should reflect the results generated by the laboratory equipment. Data related to the medication provided to a particular patient should reflect the actual date, time, and medication administered. The accuracy of the data placed in the health record depends on a number of factors, including:

- The patient's physical health and emotional state at the time the data were collected
- The provider's interviewing skills
- The provider's recording skills
- The availability of the patient's clinical history
- The dependability of the automated equipment
- The reliability of the electronic communications media

Accessibility

Data accessibility means that the data are easily obtainable. The following factors affect the accessibility of health record data and information:

- Whether previous health records are available when and where they are needed
- Whether dictation equipment is accessible and working properly
- Whether transcription of dictation is accurate, timely, and readily available to healthcare providers
- Whether computer data-entry devices are working properly and readily available to healthcare providers

Comprehensiveness

Data comprehensiveness refers to the fact that all the required data elements are included in the health record. In essence, comprehensiveness means that the record is complete. In both paper- and computer-based systems, having a complete health record is critical to the organization's ability to provide excellent patient care and to meet all regulatory, legal, and reimbursement requirements. In general, the health record must include the following data elements:

- Patient identification
- Consents for treatment
- Problem list
- Diagnoses
- Clinical history
- Diagnostic test results
- Treatments and outcomes
- Conclusions and follow-up requirements

Consistency

Data consistency refers to the reliability of the data. Reliable data do not change no matter how many times or in how many ways they are stored, processed, or displayed. Data values are consistent when the value of any given data element is the same across applications and systems. Related data items also should be reliable. For example, the clinical history for a male patient would never include a hysterectomy as a past surgical procedure.

Legitimate documentation inconsistencies do occur in health records. Any given health record may contain numerous references to the patient's diagnosis in terms of:

- The admitting diagnosis
- The diagnostic impression upon physical examination
- The postoperative diagnosis
- The pathology diagnosis
- The discharge diagnosis

Any inconsistencies among the various types of diagnoses would be legitimate. The different diagnoses incorporate the results of tests and findings unavailable at the time the previous documentation took place.

In other instances, however, data inconsistencies in the health record are unacceptable. For example, a nursing assessment might indicate that the patient is deaf when there is no documentation by the physician that the patient's hearing is compromised. Another unacceptable inconsistency occurs when different healthcare providers use different terminology. For example, different providers might use the words *cyst*, *lesion*, and *abscess* interchangeably in documenting a skin condition for the same patient. Such inconsistencies create difficulties for other caregivers and can be very confusing to external users of the health record.

Currency

Data currency and data timeliness refer to the requirement that healthcare data be up-to-date and recorded at or near the time of the event or observation. Because care and treatment rely on accurate and current data, an essential characteristic of data quality is the timeliness of the documentation or data entry.

Definition

Data definition refers to the meaning of the data and information documented in the health record. For information to be meaningful, it must be pertinent. Further, users of the data must understand what the data mean and represent. Every data element should have a clear definition and a range of acceptable values.

Granularity

Data granularity is another data quality characteristic that needs to be considered when establishing data definitions. It requires that the attributes and values of data be defined at the correct level of detail. For example, numerical values for laboratory results should be recorded to the appropriate decimal place as required for the meaningful interpretation of test results.

Precision

Data precision is the term used to describe expected data values. As part of data definition, the acceptable values or value ranges for each data element must be defined. For example, a precise data definition related to gender would include three values: male, female, and unknown. Precise data definition yields accurate data collection. In paper-based health records, much of the documentation and data are collected in narrative format and it is difficult to apply the concept of data precision to narrative text. The movement toward computer-based patient records provides the perfect opportunity to improve data precision in health records.

Relevancy

Data relevancy refers to the usefulness of the data in the health record. The reason for collecting the data element must be clear to ensure the relevancy of the data collected. Additionally, the collection instrument should be tested to validate its use (Teslow 2007, 145). For example, nursing documentation is often lengthy, and physicians and other caregivers may not have sufficient time to review it. Therefore, data users may request changes to ensure that the data are useful to them.

Approaches to Controlling Data Quality

There are many approaches to managing the quality of care in today's healthcare environment. Over the years, quality monitoring has taken on many names and methodologies. Different terms and methodologies have been used to attempt to assess and manage data quality. The term *quality assurance (QA) monitoring* has been used and typically consisted of quarterly studies performed on existing problems and issues. Although this approach was a good start, later variations such as total quality improvement attempted to view quality improvement as an ongoing process. Occurrence screens were used to identify a set number of happenings, such as deaths within 24 hours of admission or single blood transfusions, which triggered an audit by a quality committee. More recent approaches to healthcare quality management include programs such as Six Sigma and the clinical value compass.

Six Sigma

Six Sigma focuses on overall quality improvement of a service or process by eliminating variables in a process to obtain a more concise standard product or output. This process differs from other quality initiatives in several essential ways. It is a business philosophy, which becomes an integral part of the organization's business strategy, unlike programs that are instituted in just one business unit or department. Because the entire organization is involved, high-level management must assume leadership roles for a Six Sigma program. The Six Sigma process is based on measured starting points and results and has strong implications for the organization's financial performance, customer satisfaction, and employee retention (Newberry and Floss 2003).

Clinical Value Compass

The clinical value compass is another data quality methodology. It is designed to link the various components, or indicators, of a process to the directions on a compass. Each point of the compass represents a different indicator, as follows:

North	Health status or function
South	Costs of care
East	Patient satisfaction
West	Clinical outcomes

The relationship between these indicators of quality can be expressed as the following equation:

$$\frac{Clinical\ Outcomes + Functional\ Status\ Outcomes + Satisfaction}{Costs\ of\ Care}$$

As a result, each involved area, such as patient care, billing, and coding, can focus on the possible solutions from a systems approach. In other words, the problem and solutions are viewed from the vantage point of how the whole process is affected rather than just looking at one or two aspects.

The diagram in figure 7.1 shows how one team used the compass approach to reduce cardiac death in postoperative patients.

Figure 7.1. The compass approach

Functional Outcomes/Quality of Life

	Q1	Q2	Q3	Q4
Physical Function: • Before • Six months after				
Bodily pain				
General health				

Clinical Outcomes

	Target	Baseline	YTD
Mortality rate	2%	4.5	2.9
Complication rate	6%	12	7
CVA	<1.5%	2	2
Post-op bleed	<1%	1.5	2

Patient Satisfaction

	Target	Baseline	YTD
Overall satisfaction	3.5	3.2	3.6
Meet patient expectations	3.5	3.0	3.4

Resource Management

	Target	Baseline	YTD
Cost per case	$6500	$7800	$6900
Length of stay	5	7.2	6.1

Clinical Processes

	Target	Baseline	YTD
Management cardiac failure (cases)	<20%	60%	35%
Early extubation	<12 hours	35%	70%
Pre-op risk assessment	100%	45%	68%

Patient Case Mix

	Baseline	YTD
% High-risk patients	35%	32%
Age (mean)	69	70
Sex (% male)	67%	64%
Volume (total)	645	460

Source: Buff and Hohmann 1999, 46.

Appendix D (pp. 175–180) contains an article on the impact of data quality on healthcare and HIM, which presents the major elements in setting up and maintaining a vigorous data quality program across multiple hospital departments. Appendix E (pp. 181–185) includes AHIMA's practice brief on data quality that provides further information on data quality management and improvement initiatives.

Summary

Accurate and complete information is both the goal and the outcome of carefully applied processes for evaluating, controlling, and monitoring the quality of healthcare data. Quality healthcare data is driving the healthcare delivery system as it is now being used in models such as CMS's "pay for performance" initiatives and directly impacts payment for services.

Data quality is a complex issue that is difficult to discuss in isolation because it is so closely connected to other areas such as compliance, quality improvement, and the audit process. Chapter 8 provides further in-depth discussion of data quality and compliance issues, and chapter 9 presents a detailed explanation of the audit process.

Chapter 8

Coding Compliance

The U.S. government has established a defined group, with oversight by the Office of the Inspector General (OIG) of the Department of Health and Human Services (HHS), to investigate areas of fraud and abuse in the healthcare industry. The OIG works with the U.S. Department of Justice, which includes the Federal Bureau of Investigation (FBI) and the U.S. Attorney's Offices, to investigate and prosecute violations of the law. These groups also work at the individual state level with private insurance carriers, states' attorneys general, state Medicaid fraud units, fiscal intermediaries, and Medicare Part B carriers to evaluate allegations of fraud and abuse.

According to the OIG, facilities should participate voluntarily in programs designed to maintain compliance with all billing and coding regulations. To assist with this process, the OIG has published compliance program guidance for several different types of healthcare entities, including hospitals. In conjunction with the Centers for Medicare and Medicaid Services (CMS), the FBI, and other federal and state agencies, the OIG works to detect fraud and abuse in the healthcare industry.

This chapter examines the programs and policies involved in ensuring coding compliance. It also describes the components of a facility compliance plan.

See appendix F (pp. 187–199) for details on how to develop an effective compliance audit process and appendix G (pp. 201–212) for sample audit worksheets specific to inpatient settings.

Recovery Audit Contractors (RAC)

One of the newest initiatives by the government to eliminate fraud and abuse and recoup incorrect payments is found in the usage of Recovery Audit Contractors (RACs). These contractors are auditing charts to identify Medicare over- and underpayments and return incorrect payments to the government. These RACs are paid based on a percentage of money they identify and collect on behalf of the government. RACs are working to identify incorrect past Medicare payments and helping to prevent future overpayments to providers (CMS n.d.b.).

RACs primarily review areas such as medical necessity, excessive/duplicate payments, and Medicare as secondary payer issues. Additional review areas will be added as RACs become nationwide in scope.

Initial Targets: Hospitals and DRGs/MS-DRGs

RACs are initially focusing on DRG payment errors, looking at claims data from as far back as calendar year 2001. Using DRG data-mining software programs, the RAC will analyze historical

Medicare Provider Analysis and Review (MEDPAR) data and identify accounts that possess the greatest potential for DRG overpayment error. Because the random account selection is not a part of the RAC demonstration program, a variety of DRGs have been targeted for review.

A list of the top DRGs include:

- Septicemia

- Wound débridement and skin graft

- Extensive OR procedure unrelated to principal diagnosis

- Circulatory disorders except AMI, with cardiac catheterization and complex diagnosis

- Respiratory system diagnosis with ventilator support

- Other respiratory system OR procedures w/CC

- OR procedure for infectious and parasitic diseases

- Respiratory neoplasms

- Nonextensive OR procedure unrelated to principal diagnosis

- Coagulation disorders

- Major small and large bowel procedures w/CC

Identified Issues

Within this group of DRGs, the RAC has identified the three DRGs with the most changes:

- Septicemia

- Wound débridement and skin graft, except hand with débridement

- Coagulation disorders

Septicemia

Physician and clinical documentation regarding bacteremia and urosepsis continue to be inpatient coding challenges. The following scenarios are responsible for the majority of RAC designated changes.

- **790.7, Bacteremia**

  Target: Principal diagnosis assignment of bacteremia when other infectious diagnosis(es) has been documented and treated. Bacteremia is defined as the presence of bacteria in the blood. It is considered an abnormal laboratory finding for coding purposes. RAC findings indicate that coders should query physicians when bacteremia and other infectious disease processes such as pneumonia, infected ulcers, and urinary tract infections (UTI) are documented and treated during the same admission.

- **599.0, Urinary tract infection**

  Target: Secondary diagnosis of UTI when the physician documents "urosepsis," but clinical and physician documentation do not support sepsis. RAC findings indicate that coders should query physicians when urosepsis is documented without conclusive evidence of clinical indicators for sepsis.

- **996.62, Line sepsis**

  Target: Secondary diagnosis of line sepsis. AHA *Coding Clinic* states that cases of patients documented with sepsis due to infected vascular access devices, catheters, or implants should have code 996.62 sequenced as principal diagnosis. Coders need to carefully review documentation and refer to AHA *Coding Clinic* to confirm appropriate sequencing guidelines.

Wound Débridement and Skin Graft

Physician documentation regarding type of débridement (that is, sharp, excisional) as well as the depth and site of all excisional wound débridement procedures must be thoroughly reviewed by coding professionals in order to report the most appropriate ICD-9-CM procedure code. The following scenarios are responsible for the majority of RAC designated changes:

- **83.39, Débridement fascia/muscle**

  ICD-9-CM procedure code 86.22, Excisional débridement, is not appropriate for coding purposes when débridement of skin, subcutaneous tissue, and fascia are performed during the same operative encounter. Coding professionals need access to complete documentation in order to properly assign débridement procedure codes.

- **81.5x, Joint replacements**

  ICD-9-CM procedure code 86.22, Excisional débridement, should not be assigned when a débridement is performed in conjunction with joint replacement and arthroplasty procedures. Débridement of joints and surrounding tissue is considered integral to joint replacement and arthroplasty procedures.

Coagulation Disorders

The 2004 third quarter AHA *Coding Clinic* provides explicit guidelines regarding the reporting of specific bleeding disorders resulting from Coumadin therapy. ICD-9-CM code 286.5, Hemorrhagic disorder secondary to circulating anticoagulants, should not be reported when the site or type of bleeding is documented by the physician. The following scenarios are responsible for the majority of RAC designated changes (Bryant 2007):

- 599.7, Hematuria

- 784.7, Epistaxis

- 578.x, GI bleeding

Fraud and Abuse

Fraud and abuse consist of the acts of providers that are deemed to have defrauded the government or abused the right to bill for services rendered. Fraudulent activity means that the provider intentionally, or with reckless disregard for the truth, filed false healthcare claims. These findings can result in civil or criminal prosecution. Erroneous claims, or abuse, are innocent billing errors that result in the minimum of return of overpayments or funds received in error.

Federal Civil False Claims Act

The Federal Civil False Claims Act (FCA) (31 USC§3729–3733) is the legislation that provides the framework for federal fraud and abuse penalties and investigations. It defines liability for anyone who knowingly files a fraudulent claim with the intention of obtaining inappropriate funds from the government. The law specifies that a claim of fraud can be made up to ten years from the date of violation.

The phrase "knew or should have known" is frequently used in conjunction with fraud and abuse. Professionals and facilities are required to adhere to all published rules and guidance. Whether they actually knew about a certain rule does not matter; if the rule was published, it should be followed.

Operation Restore Trust

Operation Restore Trust is a program set up by the OIG as a means of combating healthcare fraud and abuse. It uses an interdisciplinary project team of federal and state government and private-sector representatives to target Medicare abuse and misuse. The project consists of federal audits by the OIG, criminal investigations by CMS, and referrals by the OIG to appropriate law enforcement officials. Civil and administrative sanction and recovery actions by the OIG and other appropriate law enforcement officials are an integral part of this plan, with actual damages that can be triple the amount of the actual inappropriate payment, and with fines of more than $11,000 per occurrence.

Other OIG Guidance for Compliance Programs

The OIG also publishes studies and recommendations for program adjustments to prevent fraud and reduce waste and abuse. Additionally, it issues special fraud alerts to notify the public and healthcare community about schemes in the provision of healthcare services. The OIG Work Plan, published each fiscal year, is a projection of the various projects to be addressed by the Office of Audit Services, Office of Evaluation and Inspections, Office of Investigations, and Office of Counsel to the Inspector General. Current work plans are available online (OIG n.d.).

The government issued the first guidance for compliance programs for hospitals in 1998. The OIG (1998) stated:

> The adoption and implementation of voluntary compliance programs significantly advance the prevention of fraud, abuse, and waste in these health care plans while at the same time furthering the fundamental mission of all hospitals, which is to provide quality care to all patients.

Seven key elements were established as guidelines for an effective compliance program. A facility should:

- Establish written policies, procedures, and standards of conduct

- Designate a chief compliance officer and appropriate committee(s)

- Provide an effective training and education program

- Develop effective communication and a process for reporting compliance issues

- Enforce the program through well-publicized disciplinary guidelines

- Audit and monitor the program

- Respond promptly to allegations by taking corrective action

The OIG published the *Supplemental Compliance Program Guidance for Hospitals* in 2005. This document also is available online.

Policies and Procedures

Definitive policies and procedures should be established and maintained to ensure that all members of the organization are following the guidelines. Comprehensive policies and procedures should include accurate coding, documentation, retention, contracts, and outsourcing. Internal coding practices should be well written, clear, and indicative that the facility follows official coding guidelines. Written coding accuracy standards and commitment should be in place to provide adequate coding resources for all coding staff. If outsourced/contract coders are utilized in the facility, they must be educated on facility policies and steps should be taken to ensure that they are following the same rules and regulations and are under the same quality measurements as hospital employed coding professionals.

Moreover, the policies and procedures should be used to identify and target possible areas of risk. Some of the most common areas of risk include:

- Unbundling or fragmenting a service by reporting separate codes for services that are included in one procedure code

- Downcoding a service in order to assign an additional code (This also can occur by inappropriately separating surgical approach from the major surgical service performed.)

Other areas of concern are as follows:

- Diagnosis or procedure misrepresentation

- Assignment of a code for a higher level of service than the service that was provided

- Diagnostic tests that are medically unnecessary

- DRG assignments including problematic areas such as pneumonia, sepsis, and respiratory failure

The policies and procedures should be communicated on a regular basis. A code of conduct should be developed that indicates a firm commitment to compliance as part of the daily routine and course of business.

Components of a Compliance Plan

The basic components of a compliance plan include designation of a compliance officer, training and education, communication strategies, auditing and monitoring activities, corrective action, and follow-up measures. In addition, mechanisms to ensure accurate and complete documentation in the health record must be in place to ensure coding and billing compliance.

Designation of Compliance Officer

In the compliance program guidance (CPG) for hospitals, the government recognized that facilities may have different needs in developing their compliance plan. The government recommends that hospitals appoint a chief compliance officer and establish a compliance committee to provide assistance and guidance, as needed.

Training and Education

Training and education is a key component of all compliance plans. There should be mandatory annual training for new hires, professional staff, and physicians. Regular meetings should be held with coding staff to ensure compliance with any new rules and regulations. Focused training sessions should take place as problematic areas are identified, and compliance should be included in all performance evaluations. Facilities should establish job descriptions and qualification requirements for professional coders and billing staff.

Communication

Communication is an essential component in all compliance plans. A mechanism must be in place for reporting perceived compliance violations. If employees feel that their complaints will be ignored or used against them in some way, they will not report problems, even though there are whistleblower laws to protect them. They need to know that compliance is not just a requirement from the government, but a part of the culture at the facility. No one member or group can be exempt from the system.

Auditing and Monitoring

Another key component of a thorough compliance program is auditing (which is discussed in greater detail in chapter 9). Auditing of the entire revenue cycle from patient service to payment should be completed on a regular basis. Some basic auditing steps include the following (OIG 2005, 4859):

- Use OIG target areas to ensure compliance with key efforts by the government to prevent fraud.

- Evaluate internal coding practices on a regular basis.

- Compare internal findings with external benchmarking practices. Frequency, scope, and size depend on organization. There is no "one size fits all" compliance plan. Plans should be developed and reviewed on an ongoing basis to ensure that they are working properly and appropriately. "The OIG strongly encourages hospitals to identify and focus their compliance efforts on those areas of potential concern or risk that are most relevant to their individual organizations."

Corrective Action and Follow-up

With any compliance issues that are identified, corrective action and follow-up must occur in a timely manner. Although the definition of "timely" may vary depending on the scope of the problem, it is commonly recommended that corrective action and follow-up happen within sixty days of the date the complaint is reported. If employees feel that their concerns are ignored, they are less likely to report possible violations in the future.

As hospitals work to maintain and promote compliance in their facilities, they should examine several areas. These include monitoring of case-mix index, comparison of coding and billing patterns, and monitoring and evaluation of denials and implementation of coding updates.

Monitor and Understand the Case-Mix Index

The case-mix index (CMI) is the average DRG weight for a set of patients for a given time period. A CMI close to 1.000 shows that the facility's patients are using approximately the same amount of resources as the average Medicare patient. A higher CMI indicates patients who are more acutely ill than the average Medicare patient. As the government monitors submitted data in the Med PAR database, a hospital with a CMI that is statistically higher than that of surrounding areas may raise concern. In the early days of fraud and abuse investigations, several hospitals with unusually high CMIs were found to have improper coding and billing practices. (See table 8.1 for a typical CMI.)

The CMI should be calculated and tracked over time to allow the facility to monitor for unusual events that have an impact on the overall CMI. For example, one or two highly weighted DRGs (such as MS-DRG 002 with a relative weight of 16.2735) will create an abnormally high CMI. If the facility in this example had one additional patient in MS-DRG 927 with a relative weight of 12.3042, the CMI would jump to 4.922. This high CMI does not accurately reflect the amount of resources used by the average patient in the facility.

Compare Utilization and Billing Patterns with National, State, and Regional Norms

A common practice is to benchmark with other facilities with similar traits, such as bed size and patient mix. This allows the hospital to evaluate its performance statistics in comparison to like hospitals and review any unusual findings.

Compare Coding and Billing Patterns Over Time

Facilities also can benchmark internally. The facility might use a simple graph to chart patterns over different time periods to determine problem areas. It also should look for areas of concern, such as an unusually high CMI or a drop in reimbursement.

Table 8.1. Example of CMI

Patient	MS-DRG	MS-DRG Weight
1	89	0.9479
2	434	1.0125
3	55	1.1213
4	478	1.9836

Total MS-DRG weight = 5.0653/4 = 1.266325.

Monitor Claims Denials and Error Reports

As much as possible, facilities should have staff dedicated to monitoring all denials and claims that are returned to provider (RTP). A simple spreadsheet, as shown in table 8.2, can be developed to monitor denials to evaluate areas for education and improvement in coding and billing practices.

Monitor Coding and DRG Changes

Facilities should monitor claims carefully in the first few months after coding changes take effect. These changes affect coding, billing, and documentation practices and should be reviewed to ensure that correct and complete claims are submitted. Some insurance companies may not have uploaded coding changes into their computer systems and may erroneously deny claims that make use of new codes.

Appeal Inappropriate Denials

As denials are being monitored, it is imperative that incorrect or inappropriate denials be appealed.

Documentation Requirements

As discussed in other chapters, documentation in the health record is key to ensuring coding and billing compliance. According to Medicare, documentation should be available to the coder at the time of coding and sufficient to support the claim. It should be timely, with dictation and transcription completed as soon as possible after discharge. An established mechanism must be in place for obtaining physician clarification when the documentation is incomplete, illegible, or ambiguous so that billing accurately reflects the services provided.

Quality Improvement Organizations

To ensure that the federal government pays only for medically necessary, appropriate, and high-quality healthcare services, CMS contracts with medical review organizations called quality improvement organizations (QIOs). These organizations were formerly known as PROs, or peer review organizations. QIOs work with hospitals and other healthcare organizations in their area to conduct studies designed to help improve quality of care for Medicare beneficiaries. The QIOs' contract with CMS is known as the Scope of Work (SOW), a document that specifies the goals and topics for review. According to Qsource (2005), for the state

Table 8.2. Example of denial spreadsheet

Reason for Denial	No. of Patients	Amount
Medical necessity	15	$4,345
Noncovered services	3	$2,356
CCI edits	5	$6,742

of Tennessee, the QIO's "approach to quality improvement focuses on patterns of care, with the primary goal of studying and improving the mainstream of care."

Hospital Payment Monitoring Program

Through the SOW, CMS has reviewed problematic DRGs over the past several years. Originally, in 1999, this program was known as the Payment Error Prevention Program (PEPP). The QIOs worked with hospitals to monitor their documentation and coding practices to ensure compliance with Medicare initiatives to prevent fraud and abuse.

Medicare Quality Initiative

Section 501(b) of the Medicare Modernization Act (MMA) requires that certain inpatient hospitals submit quality data to the secretary of the HHS on a set of indicators, as established by the secretary as of November 1, 2003, in order to receive a full-payment update. Hospitals that do not submit data in the form and manner specified will have their payment update reduced by 2 percentage points. The Requirements for Hospital Reporting of Quality Data for Annual Payment Update is available online from Quality Net (n.d.).

Specific Coding Problem Areas

Based on studies of coding patterns, the OIG is able to target specific problem areas that result in inaccurate coding and payment. Pneumonias constitute one such problem area; septicemia and related conditions are another.

Pneumonias

The OIG has performed several studies relating to the issues of pneumonia coding because of patterns indicating inaccurate coding and payment for bacterial cases of pneumonia. Clinically, there are many different types of pneumonia. Code 486, pneumonia, organism unspecified, should be used only when the health record does not identify the causative organism. Therefore, it is important that the coder review the entire medical record and possibly query the physician to determine whether a more specific code can be used. Even when the coder finds a positive culture in the laboratory findings, such as for *Klebsiella pneumoniae,* this cannot be coded as Pneumonia due to Klebsiella pneumoniae without confirmation from the physician of a cause-and-effect relationship.

Viral pneumonia is highly contagious and typically affects the trachea and bronchi of the lungs. Pneumococcal pneumonia is caused by pneumococcal/streptococcus pneumoniae bacteria. Clinical indicators include documentation of pleural friction and chest x-ray showing consolidation from pus. Other bacterial pneumonias caused by agents such as *Klebsiella, Pseudomonas,* and *Streptococcus* are common in the adult population and are usually identified through Gram staining of sputum. Because of differences in the quality of a sputum culture and the possibility of contamination as the sputum travels through the airway, *Coding Clinic for ICD-9-CM* states that a Gram-positive cocci finding should not be coded as the cause of bacterial pneumonia without further clinical findings and documentation by the physician.

Coding Clinic guidelines for coding Gram-negative pneumonia include findings such as worsening of cough, dyspnea, reduction of oxygen level, fever, purulent sputum, and patchy infiltration on chest x-ray. It may appear as a complication of surgery, trauma, or chronic illnesses, or in chronic obstructive pulmonary disease (COPD) and immunosuppressive drug therapy patients.

Septicemia

Another problem identified by the OIG is that of incorrect coding of sepsis. Clinically, sepsis may look similar to a urinary tract infection, which is often documented as urosepsis, and there is a large difference in DRG payment. It is very important that the coder understand findings in the health record in order to code the diagnoses appropriately.

In the past, sepsis and septicemia were coded the same, but over the past several years, the "systemic inflammatory response syndrome-sepsis-severe sepsis-septic shock continuum" has been established. The patient first may exhibit signs of bacteremia. Bacteremia is the presence of bacteria in the blood and is coded to 790.7. It can lead to sepsis but is not necessarily the same thing. The coder should query the physician, especially when bacteremia is found with two or fewer signs of sepsis. Transient bacteremia may occur in other diseases such as pneumonia, but if it lasts over several days, it may mean that there is an infected vessel or heart valve.

Septicemia, code 038.X, is defined as "an infectious disease due to the accumulation and persistence of bacteria and/or their toxins in the blood and marked by high fever, shaking chills, prostration, and if untreated, hypotension, shock and death" (Channel 2008, 282). It is a systemic disease.

Systemic Inflammatory Response Syndrome (995.9x)

Systemic inflammatory response syndrome (SIRS) is considered a major complication consisting of the body's reaction to infection or trauma. It includes systemic inflammation, rapid heart rate and respiration, and an elevated white blood cell count that may develop into multiorgan dysfunction (MOD) or failure (Channel 2008, 661). Sepsis codes are sequenced after the code for the underlying infection, such as septicemia.

Sepsis (995.91)

The definition of sepsis is a SIRS reaction plus documented infection. Common symptoms include mental status changes, especially in the elderly patient; oliguria; and sustained hypotension.

Severe Sepsis (995.92)

Severe sepsis consists of sepsis plus end-organ dysfunction. It may include multiple-organ failure, including kidney and respiratory failure, encephalopathy, or critical illness myopathy or polyneuropathy. Each organ dysfunction should be coded along with the severe sepsis code. If there is question in the documentation whether the organ dysfunction is or is not from the sepsis, then query the physician. This patient typically requires extensive treatment with high-cost medications such as Xigris, which is separately reported as a procedure code for add-on payment.

Septic Shock (785.52)

The last phase of the continuum is septic shock, which is defined as "sepsis with sepsis-induced hypotension despite fluid resuscitation and inadequate tissue perfusion (failure of peripheral circulation) (Channel 2008, 599). Many patients do not recover when they reach this point in the continuum.

Coding Guidance for Septicemia

According to *Coding Clinic for ICD-9-CM*, a negative blood culture does not mean the patient does not have septicemia. If clinical signs substantiate the diagnosis, however, the physician must show a clear link between the culture findings and the diagnosis.

Treatment for sepsis usually includes high dosages of IV antibiotics; thus, if a patient has been on antibiotics prior to the blood culture, this may account for a negative (normal) appearing result. Clinical indicators include positive blood cultures, white blood cell (WBC) count greater than 14,000, fever, and oliguria. When the term *urosepsis* is used, the physician should be queried to determine the proper diagnosis. The main problem identified in government DRG validation studies included "clinical findings in the chart not specified/verified by physician"; thus, it is very important that coders review the chart carefully and query the physician to ensure correct coding. Facilities should continue to review cases in MS-DRGs for sepsis and septicemia, especially those with a short length of stay, and to continue to educate physicians on updated terminology to assist with proper coding. The coding professional should also carefully review the chart for mechanical ventilation, as patients with 96 or more hours of mechanical ventilation tend to stay in the hospital longer and utilize more resources. *Coding Clinic for ICD-9-CM* and *ICD-9-CM Official Guidelines for Coding and Reporting* should be reviewed for more detailed information as noted below in the chapter-specific guidelines:

The coding of SIRS, sepsis, and severe sepsis requires a minimum of two codes: A code for the underlying cause (such as infection or trauma) and a code from subcategory 995.9 Systemic inflammatory response syndrome (SIRS). These codes are detailed below.

(i)   The code for the underlying cause (such as infection or trauma) must be sequenced before the code from subcategory 995.9 Systemic inflammatory response syndrome (SIRS).

(ii)   Sepsis and severe sepsis require a code for the systemic infection (038.xx, 112.5, etc.) and either code 995.91, Sepsis, or 995.92, Severe sepsis. If the causal organism is not documented, assign code 038.9, Unspecified septicemia.

(iii)   Severe sepsis requires additional code(s) for the associated acute organ dysfunction(s).

(iv)   If a patient has sepsis with multiple organ dysfunctions, follow the instructions for coding severe sepsis.

(v)   Either the term sepsis or SIRS must be documented to assign a code from subcategory 995.9.

(vi)   See Section I.C.17.g), Injury and poisoning, for information regarding systemic inflammatory response syndrome (SIRS) due to trauma/burns and other non-infectious processes.

Due to the complex nature of sepsis and severe sepsis, some cases may require querying the provider prior to assignment of the codes. (NCHS 2007, 15).

According to Official Coding Guidelines, the codes should be sequenced based on whether the patient had evidence of sepsis on admission and should follow the definition of principal diagnosis. The instructional note under subcategory 995.9 instructs to assign the underlying condition first.

- Note: The term *urosepsis* is nonspecific. If it is the only term documented, only code 599.0 should be assigned based on the default for the term in the ICD-9-CM index, in addition to the code for the causal organism, if known.

- For patients with severe sepsis, the code for the systemic infection (038.xx, 112.5, and so forth) or trauma should be sequenced first, followed by either code 995.92, Systemic inflammatory response syndrome due to infectious process with organ dysfunction, or code 995.94, Systemic inflammatory response syndrome due to noninfectious process with organ dysfunction. Codes for the specific organ dysfunction also should be assigned.

- If septic shock is documented, it is necessary to code first the initiating systemic infection or trauma and then either code 995.92 or 995.94, followed by code 785.52, Septic shock.

The QIOs have developed a workbook that includes forms to assist hospitals with reviewing charts for appropriate coding on topics such as sepsis and pneumonias. The materials are offered free of charge from Qsource (2005).

Summary

Because hospitals are paid for inpatient care based primarily on codes, it is vital that coders have a clear understanding of appropriate and compliant coding. Facilities throughout the country have had to make repayments to the government because of improper coding, sequencing, and billing of diagnosis and procedure codes. Most facilities have not set out to defraud the government purposely but, rather, have made mistakes because of a lack of policies, procedures, and appropriate compliance training. Compliance should not be another buzzword; rather, it should be part of a culture in which all members of the healthcare team work together to ensure that complete and accurate documentation leads to correct and adequate payment for services.

Applying the Guidelines

The following case examples are designed to increase the reader's understanding of and ability to select appropriate principal and secondary diagnoses. The correct answers are found at the end of the chapter.

Case 8.1

History of Present Illness

The patient is a 54-year-old black male with a five-day history of feeling ill. When his daughter went by his house today to check on him, she found him clammy with a fever and very disoriented. Lab results in the ER showed UTI, probable sepsis, renal insufficiency. BUN, Creatinine elevated. WBC count was 23,000. The patient was admitted for treatment of probable urinary sepsis.

Findings While in the Hospital

WBCs fell during hospitalization to 9,000. Urine culture grew *E. coli;* blood cultures also grew *E. coli.* No other abnormalities noted.

Hospital Course

The patient was started on IV fluid rehydration; electrolytes improved throughout stay. He was started on IV antibiotics and switched to oral antibiotics the day of discharge. The patient was discharged to his daughter's care at her home until he gets back on his feet.

Answer:

Principal Diagnosis: _____

Secondary Diagnoses: _____

Questions for Physician: _____

Case 8.2

DISCHARGE DIAGNOSES: UTI, Urosepsis, Pneumonia

HISTORY: The patient is a 74-year-old male who complains of fever, chills, and not feeling well generally. Urine culture had been done the day prior to admission due to frequent UTI problems and was positive for *E. coli,* so he was started on Cipro. Admission urinalysis showed a large number of white cells and nitrate. WBC count was 14,000. Sputum cultures were positive for *Klebsiella pneumoniae.*

HOSPITAL COURSE: The patient was started on IV fluids to rehydrate him and Ancef added to his Cipro meds. Urine cultures continued to have increased white cells. Blood cultures taken on the second day were normal. Chest cleared to normal by discharge.

Answer:

Principal Diagnosis: _____

Secondary Diagnoses: _____

Questions for Physician: _____

Answers to Case Studies

Case 8.1

Principal Diagnosis: The physician states "probable sepsis" and all clinical evidence (blood cultures, mental status changes) points to that as the main reason for admission. Underlying cause (such as *E. coli* septicemia) would need to be verified. Since the patient has renal insufficiency, the coder needs to query the physician to see if this is more appropriately coded to severe sepsis. Since official coding guidelines do allow for coding "probable" at present, it is technically correct to code sepsis; however, a query to the physician would be indicated to obtain the most appropriate information. Urinary sepsis codes to 599.0; however, it appears the doctor may mean sepsis, which would be coded to 038.9, 995.91. The coder should query for cause and effect relationship of positive blood culture *E. coli* to sepsis for 038.42 and would need more information from the chart to determine if the patient had acute renal failure and the 995.92 severe sepsis with organ dysfunction for acute renal failure (584.9).

Secondary Diagnoses: UTI 599.0
E. coli 041.4
Patient was started on IV fluid rehydration. Clarify with the physician: Is dehydration a codeable diagnosis?

MS-DRG Grouping Issues: If this case is grouped with the UTI as the principal diagnosis, it falls into MS-DRG 690, Kidney and Urinary Tract Infection without MCC, which is weighted 0.8000 and has an approximate payment of $5043.46. If the physician query justifies the septicemia as the principal diagnosis, it groups to MS-DRG 872, Septicemia without Mechanical Ventilation Greater than 96 hours, without MCC. The weight is 1.3783 with approximate payment at $8689.25.

Case 8.2

Principal Diagnosis: The coder needs to verify in the record and query the physician as to the main reason for admission. Nonspecific diagnosis of urosepsis needs to be clarified; it could mean urinary sepsis (coded as UTI, 599.0) or sepsis. Blood cultures were negative, but this does not preclude a diagnosis of sepsis according to *Coding Clinic*. Also, sputum culture grew out *Klebsiella*. The coder should verify that documentation supports that as the cause for the pneumonia (482.0) by querying the physician. This case could be "multiple conditions present on admission" because it appears that either the pneumonia or UTI/sepsis could be the chief reason for admission.

Secondary Diagnoses: UTI 599.0
E. Coli 041.4

MS-DRG Grouping Issues: The order of the diagnoses and level of specificity provided through the query process can have a tremendous impact on correct reimbursement in this case. After querying the physician, if the UTI is found to meet the definition of principal diagnosis, with the pneumonia due to *Klebsiella* as secondary (counting as an MCC), it groups to MS-DRG 689 with a weight of 1.0587 and an approximate payment of $6674.40.

If septicemia is determined to be the principal diagnosis, MS-DRG 871 is weighted at 1.7484 with an approximate payment of $8989.25.

If the *Klebsiella pneumonia* is the principal diangosis with a secondary diagnosis of UTI instead of septicemia, the correct MS-DRG is 178 with a weight of 1.5636 and an approximate payment of $9857.46. If *Klebsiella pneumonia* is the principal diagnosis with both UTI and sepsis/septicemia are coded as secondary diagnoses, the MS-DRG 177 would be assigned which has a weight of 1.8444 and approximate payment of $11,627.71.

MS-DRG	Relative Weight	Approximate Payment
689	1.0587	$6674.40
871	1.7484	$8989.24
178	1.5636	$9857.46
177	1.8444	$11,627.71

Chapter 9

The Health Record Auditing Process

In simplest terms, an inpatient health record audit is a methodical examination and review of a hospital's coding and billing processes. This chapter discusses the types of code audits, the different methods for reviewing them, and how to design and implement a code audit.

Plan of Action for Setting Up or Updating a Health Record Auditing Process

When establishing or updating an auditing process, the healthcare facility should develop a plan of action based on consideration of the following issues:

- What does the facility want to accomplish with the auditing program? What are its goals and objectives?

- What resources are needed in terms of personnel, time, finances, and so forth?

- What should the time frame be? One big audit per quarter? Several ongoing audit and monitoring projects?

- What forms are needed? Several companies and textbooks provide audit samples, or the facility can create its own forms.

- How can the facility achieve buy-in from staff, physicians, and administration? The more people feel ownership of a program, the more likely they are to participate willingly.

During the audit, the reviewers should look for patterns and trends, strengths and weaknesses, and problems that might be uncovered during the auditing process. They also should have access to all documents and be able to work independently so that they can remain objective in all areas. With strong commitment from the facility's administration, the reviewers should be able to obtain a true picture of its compliance program without worrying about "stepping on toes" or feeling that a particular group of people is off limits or exempt from compliance activities.

Compliance Program Guidance

The Hospital Payment Monitoring Program (HPMP) and its precursor, the Payment Error Protection Program (PEPP), have resulted in a number of excellent methods and structures for coding and reimbursement evaluation. Health information management (HIM) professionals can look to resources provided by quality improvement organizations (QIOs) (and the earlier peer review organizations), under contract with government agencies for reliable means to improve processes and minimize the risk of noncompliance.

An effective auditing and monitoring program shows that standards and procedures are current and accurate and that the compliance program is being carried out effectively. In its 2005 Supplemental Compliance Program Guidance for Hospitals, the Office of the Inspector General (OIG) identified the following areas of potential risk for hospitals that should be incorporated into the auditing portion of their compliance programs (OIG 2005):

- *Submission of accurate claims and information:* Ensuring that claims are accurate and complete remains the largest area of risk for hospitals. Documentation must support all services provided and billed and show that the service is "reasonable and necessary" for treatment of the patient's condition.

- *Referral statutes:* The physician self-referral law (Stark) prohibits hospitals from submitting claims for services provided as part of a "prohibited financial relationship." This includes certain joint ventures and compensation relationships with physicians, such as recruitment or discounts.

- *Payments to reduce or limit services:* This includes inappropriate gain-sharing or cost-sharing procedures whereby the physician may have an incentive to reduce or limit services to a beneficiary.

- *The Emergency Medical Treatment and Labor Act (EMTALA):* EMTALA was established to prevent hospitals from inappropriately transferring patients who are unstable or in active labor. Documentation must substantiate that appropriate screening and approval was done prior to any transfer or referral to other healthcare facilities.

- *Quality of care:* Providing substandard care can be viewed as a form of fraudulent activity even when services are billed correctly. Hospitals are obligated to review the quality of services provided by their medical staff and employees for all patients, not just Medicare or Medicaid patients.

- *Relationships with federal health beneficiaries:* Hospitals must take care to avoid inappropriate incentives to patients by providing any prohibited services such as gifts or free transportation.

- *HIPAA Privacy and Security Rules:* The facility must ensure strict compliance with the rules governing the privacy and security of patient information established by the Health Insurance Portability and Accountability Act (HIPAA) of 1996.

- *Medicare or Medicaid billing:* The facility must ensure that it is not billing Medicare or Medicaid in excess of usual charges.

Types of Audits

The main types of audits are coding audits, claims audits, and audits of policies and procedures. Some organizations choose to review coding accuracy and conduct claims review separately. Coding accuracy requires individual record assessment whereas some aspects of claims review are based on aggregate data analysis.

Coding Audits

All facilities should perform coding audits on at least a quarterly basis with the understanding that compliance must be an ongoing process. A comprehensive review should include a sample of all physicians, types of patients, and common diagnoses and procedures. The internal auditor should act as an external auditor by avoiding assumptions, and the record should reflect enough documentation to substantiate any diagnosis or procedure performed. A summary of the results should be prepared and shared with coders, physicians, and administration, as needed. Any coding assessment should include verification that the codes selected for cases are the same codes reported for any external purpose, such as reimbursement from a third party.

Claims Audits

Claims audits are performed on a regular basis to ensure that claims are processed in accordance with required healthcare program and billing regulations. In addition, they are done to determine the completeness of medical record documentation in supporting the services billed. Audits or chart reviews also help to verify that the codes selected are exactly the same as those submitted to the insurance company.

Audits of Policies and Procedures

The organization's compliance plan, coding policy, and other policies and procedures should be reviewed at least annually. Adherence to the hospital's compliance plan should be audited and monitored periodically to ensure its effectiveness. The procedure manual should not have to be dusted off when it comes down from the shelf; rather, it should be a fluid, current document that is frequently used by staff as a reference tool.

Methods for Review

The method used to review code audits may vary depending on whether an initial diagnostic audit or a focused review based on a specific problem area is being performed. One common approach is to use published statistical reports for comparison. For example, *The Medicare DRG Handbook*, published by Solucient, could be used for this purpose. This manual is compiled from the MEDPAR file and summarizes key findings by the top fifty highest-volume DRGs, which constitutes a large percentage of the total discharges of more than 500 total DRGs. Any organization's data can be compared and contrasted with the key findings in this manual. While this book and others like it are still available, with the implementation of the MS-DRG system in FY 2008, facilities should monitor data carefully. As data is compiled utilizing the MS-DRG groupings, updated publications will be available. The AHIMA book *Analyzing the Impact of MS-DRGs* (Hyde and Spencer 2008) is designed to assist facilities in converting their facility's top 10/high risk/high volumes DRG data into MS-DRG data and performing audits based on that facility-specific information.

Inpatient coding quality measures include (Wilson 2008):

- Accurate ICD-9-CM code assignment to the principal and secondary (additional) diagnoses.

- Accurate ICD-9-CM code assignment to the principal and other procedures.

- Accurate DRG assignment for inpatient reimbursement.

- Accurate present on admission (POA) indicator for all ICD-9-CM diagnosis codes, excluding codes published on the exempt list.

- Accurate patient status (discharge disposition) assignment.

Two types of record review methods are used in inpatient settings: the record method and the code method.

Record Method

The record method considers each incorrectly coded record to be one error. There are several advantages to this method, including:

- It is commonly used in hospitals, which allows for benchmarking.

- It permits the reviewer to track errors by case type.

- It enables the reviewer to relate productivity to quality errors on a case basis.

The disadvantages to the record method include the following:

- It oversimplifies the type of records coded because it does not recognize the coder's identification of codes that should be reported.

- It identifies neither the number of secondary diagnoses nor procedures missed by the coder.

Code Method

The code method compares the total number of codes identified by the coder to the total number of possible codes that should have been reported. The advantages to the code method include the following:

- It recognizes the coder's ability to identify all codes.

- It weighs the more resource-intensive cases by code.

- It better identifies the kinds of errors the coder is making (for example, omission of secondary diagnoses or missed sequencing).

The disadvantages to the code method include the following:

- It is difficult to compare results with benchmarking activities of other organizations.

- It does not assist with the diagnosis of case-type coder educational needs.

Benchmarking best practices shows that the code-on-code methodology is a more accurate way to calculate error rate. "A coding error is any code that is revised, added, or deleted" (Wilson 2008). These are defined as:

- **Revised code:** Revised codes are counted as *one error* or *one revision* when the *condition* or *procedure* being validated requires any of the following types of code changes: Resequencing such as moving a secondary diagnosis or procedure to principal diagnosis or principal procedure; deleting one code and revising the second code to report the combination code for the condition or procedure (300.00 and 311 being validated, auditor deletes one code and revises second code to 300.4); revising one code to more accurately reflect the condition (496 being validated, auditor revises to 491.21) or procedure (45.13 being validated, auditor revises to 45.16) or other similar revision or resequencing to the code(s) being validated.

- **Added code:** Code not reported by coder but meets secondary diagnosis or procedure reporting guidelines. Auditor counts one error for each code added, for example, adding a diagnosis or procedure code to more completely reflect a condition or procedure (for example, the auditor adds 995.91 to sepsis; adds a manifestation code; or adds a "code also" procedure code as in the case of a type of bearing surface 00.74–00.77).

- **Deleted code:** Code reported by coder but does not meet secondary diagnosis or procedure reporting guidelines. Auditor counts one error for each code deleted.

A correct code is any code that is not revised, added, or deleted.

Reviewed codes are the total number of codes reviewed (after auditing): correct codes + coding errors (+ revised codes + added codes – deleted codes).

NOTE: Do *NOT* count the number of codes coded by the coder for the denominator. Count the number of codes validated by the auditor as "reviewed codes" for the denominator.

Design and Implementation of a Coding Audit

The design and implementation of a coding audit begins with goal setting, which includes establishing an ongoing monitor for identifying problems or opportunities to improve the quality of coded data for inpatient and outpatient cases. The plan should clarify monitoring and evaluation methods. The appropriate supervisor will be responsible for identifying problems that relate to coding issues based on analysis of the review results.

Audit Team

Facilities should consider having an audit team made up of members from several key departments, including HIM/coding, billing, finance, compliance, and case management. The team should be educated on aspects of auditing and the billing cycle to ensure that all members are aware of the important role each department plays in revenue cycle management. Training should include an overview of the coding process, as well as discussion of payment systems, *ICD-9-CM Official Guidelines for Coding and Reporting*, and facility-specific policies and procedures.

Sample Review Size

The type of review being planned determines the sample size. A 200-case review is usually adequate for an initial diagnostic review. Focused MS-DRG reviews may be limited to only 10 to 15 percent of the cases, or 100 percent of the cases may be pulled. Of course, the larger the sample size, the greater the confidence in the results. The number of cases to pull for a coder-specific review depends on the number of cases the individual codes. For an annual review of coding quality for a specific coder, fifty cases should be pulled for full-time staff and twenty-five for part-time staff.

Although there is no absolute correct number of charts to audit, the industry standard is approximately 10 to 25 charts per provider. For many years, the Joint Commission recommended that studies include five percent or thirty charts, whichever is greater. The hardest part of auditing is picking a good sample that is reflective of the entire population. Several software packages and auditing books are available to help establish a good (fair) sample. One way to establish an appropriate sample is to pick every "nth" chart, such as every tenth chart coded, every fifth surgical case, and so forth. Additionally, the facility might select an occurrence to study and have coders, transcriptionists, and/or chart-processing staff keep a log whenever an event occurs. For example, in the past, sepsis stays of less than three days was referred to as occurrence screening.

Recommendations from the AHIMA e-HIM workgroup are illustrated in figure 9.1.

Figure 9.1. Inpatient coding quality audits

Type of Review:

Established coder: Quarterly or biannual.

New hire coder: Baseline or 100 percent of reviews during Orientation and Training until passing to an established coder.

- Type of review may be further refined by pre-bill and post-bill.

  Note: Coding accuracy is calculated the same for pre-bill or post-bill reviews regardless of the DRG billed.

- Type of review may be further refined by representative sample or focused sample.

  —*Representative sample* is a selection of records at random with no pre-identified DRG, documentation, coding, or coder issue.

  —A *focused review* is a selection of records with a pre-identified DRG, documentation, coding, or coder issue.

Record Sampling Methodology:

- **Timeframe**

  —*For quarterly,* the three-month timeframe not previously reviewed.

  —*For biannual,* the six-month timeframe not previously reviewed.

Note: The records selected should occur after the coder education date of the last audit. In addition, the most recent discharges should be selected.

Number of Records

Representative sample: Random selection of 2% of the required productivity standards per patient type coded (including maternity and newborn if applicable) by the coder for the timeframe selected for the review (quarterly or biannual).

Note: This random selection may be selected by first picking a number 0 through 9. For example, 5 is selected, then consecutively select every account number ending in 5 per patient type as part of your sample until you have the total records selected for your sample size.

Focused sample: 30 records or all records in the timeframe if less than 30 available.

Source: Wilson 200,8 5–6.

Recommended Topics for Auditing

Although facilities vary according to patient mix, problems identified, and so forth, certain topics lend themselves to auditing. Some recommended topics for auditing include:

- OIG work plan
- Fraud alerts
- Top 10 surgeries
- Top 10 MS-DRGs
- High-volume, high-risk procedures
- Top 10 denials
- Top 10 services provided
- Use of most specific code available
- Data-entry errors
- All orders written and signed by physician
- Review of assignment codes and modifier usage
- All tests ordered were actually performed
- MS-DRG payments
- Inpatient outliers
- Consecutive inpatient stays
- Medical necessity
- Restraint-related deaths
- Coronary artery stents

Focused Coding Reviews

When the initial diagnostic review has been completed, focused reviews based on specific problem areas should be planned. Topics identified for the focused reviews also may be based on controversial issues identified through *Coding Clinic for ICD-9-CM*. Some potential topics for the focused reviews include:

- Surgical complications
- Obstetrical complications
- Error MS-DRGs
- Diabetes mellitus
- Dehydration as principal diagnosis
- Gastrointestinal bleeding
- OIG-identified paired/families of MS-DRGs
- Recent issues identified by external review agencies and/or professional journals

In *Benchmarking to Improve Coding Accuracy and Productivity*, Wilson discusses common target areas for inpatient coding audits (2008):

1. Review Septic patients in comparison to Urinary Tract Infection patients.

2. Review Complex Pneumonia patients in comparison to Community Acquired pneumonia. For example, some organizations were placed under focused review by the OIG for upcoding complex pneumonia based on clinical indications such as: an elderly, nursing home patient who has a gastrostomy (PEG) tube and a fever. According to the American Hospital Association (AHA) Coding Clinic, coders can only code from physician documentation.

3. Review patient status (discharge disposition) code assignments on all records selected for a coding review. The patient status (discharge disposition) code is the code assignment for the destination of the patient at discharge. It will save the coding quality manager time if, while the manager is performing coding reviews, the discharge disposition code is also verified.

An MS-DRG example audit would be to analyze specific documentation of congestive heart failure (CHF). Run a report of principal and secondary ICD-9-CM codes 428.0 (CHF) by physician. This will enable the coding manager to determine which physicians need education regarding the appropriate documentation of heart failure.

The Review Process

For a code audit, the coder first reviews the medical record to ensure that the diagnosis billed as principal meets the official Uniform Hospital Discharge Data Set (UHDDS) definition. The principal diagnosis is defined as the reason determined after study to have occasioned the admission of the patient to the hospital for care. It must have been present on admission, been a principal reason for admission, and received treatment or evaluation during the stay. When several diagnoses meet all these requirements, any of them may be selected as principal diagnosis. If the principal diagnosis was chosen incorrectly, the correct diagnosis must be determined. If this can be done using coding conventions and guidelines, the attending physician does not need to be consulted. However, if the documentation in the medical record is unclear, the attending physician should be asked to clarify. If any changes affect the MS-DRG, the case will need to be rebilled. Physician clarification should be included as an addendum to the medical record that supports the code selection. The problem and its source should be identified and corrective action to prevent a recurrence implemented.

Identifying Data Quality Evaluation Indicators for Inpatient Cases

The error types identified during review will fall into the categories listed below:

- Incorrect selection of principal diagnosis

- Principal diagnosis not supported by documentation in the health record

- Substitution of a secondary diagnosis for the correct principal diagnosis

- Miscoding

- Incomplete identification of all secondary diagnoses

- Principal procedure not selected or coded correctly

- Other procedures not coded correctly

See AHIMA's *Benchmarking to Improve Coding Accuracy and Productivity* for the survey and analysis (Wilson 2008).

Reporting the Review Results

A summary of the results should be prepared and shared with coders, physicians, and other healthcare providers, including nursing staff, physical and occupational therapists, respiratory therapists, others whose documentation may have been reviewed, and administration, as needed. Often one of the hardest parts of auditing and monitoring is that of presenting the findings to the team, but this is an essential piece of the compliance program. Most physicians and staff want to know the results of audits and recommendations on how to improve their processes.

Findings should be presented as a pictorial display, using bar graphs or pie charts as appropriate. When poor or inadequate documentation is found to be a key factor causing the coding error or when physicians consistently do not respond to query requests, it is important to share these findings with the physician. If education does not help to alleviate the problem, it may be necessary to report this to the chief of the deparment/chief of the medical staff and/or administration of the facility.

If the coding staff includes a large number of clinical coding specialists, a rotating schedule should be established to include all coders on an annual basis. The review schedule depends on the number of coders and the identified problems. Initially, a large study including all coding staff and representative common diagnoses and procedures should be conducted.

Taking Action

When a problem is identified, it is important to take appropriate action in a timely manner. It is likewise important to remember that the auditing process is a learning process, not a police action. A compliant culture is one in which the information discovered during the review is used to train employees and educate physicians and to identify resources and training needs for the future, with the ultimate goal of making the billing process more accurate and effective.

Appendix F (pp. 187–199) provides further details on how to develop an effective compliance audit process. Sample audit forms and tools can be found in appendix G (pp. 201–212).

Summary

The health record audit process allows a facility to systematically examine and review its coding and billing processes with the goal of identifying and correcting problem areas. Regular health record audits provide the foundation for coding and corporate compliance.

Exercises

Under the inpatient prospective payment system (IPPS), health record documentation must support the principal diagnosis and principal procedure designations, as well as all other diagnoses and procedures submitted on the claim. Documentation should also support present on admission (POA) indicator assignment when required.

For each coding problem in this section, the documentation should be reviewed to identify:

1. The principal diagnosis (PDX) as defined as the reason, after study, that caused the patient to be admitted to the hospital. The coding professional must remember that this may not be the diagnosis listed first by the physician.

2. Other diagnoses and procedures that meet secondary reporting requirements

3. The principal procedure

4. Information to be clarified with the attending physician in a query

In selecting diagnoses or procedures for coding, the coder should assume that the documentation provided is the only documentation available. If no documentation is available to indicate a condition affecting treatment or length of stay, do not report this condition.

On the job, the coder may review other sections of the health record and consult the attending physician, if necessary, for assistance in sequencing and code selection. In the following problems, however, the discharge summary is the only documentation available to the coder. Answers for each sequencing or coding problem must be based solely on the *ICD-9-CM Official Guidelines for Coding and Reporting* including sequencing guidelines, ICD-9-CM coding conventions and principles, and AHA ICD-9-CM *Coding Clinic* advice. The attending physician has approved the diagnoses as listed in the discharge summary.

Exercise 1

History of Present Illness: This 72-year-old female presented to the ENT Clinic complaining of her current epistaxis for seven days prior to admission. The bleeding usually occurred from the right nostril. She had no prior history of epistaxis and denied any rhinorrhea, congestion, or anosmia. On admission she also complained of weakness. Four days prior to admission, she was noted to have a hematocrit of 35, and the night before her admission, she was found to have a hematocrit of 29 at an outside hospital. Her past medical history was significant for rheumatoid arthritis. Her past surgical history: status post bilateral knee replacement and right hip replacement. Medications at the time of admission included Prednisone 2 mg po bid. and aspirin, six to eight per day for the past several months. Allergies: none.

Physical Examination: On physical exam at the time of her admission, she was afebrile. Her blood pressure was 114/70 and her pulse was 92. Examination of the head and neck was significant for nasal cavities, which were without lesions and without physical bleeding sites. The remainder of the head and neck examination was within normal limits. Her neck was normal with no jugular venous distention. The lungs were clear. The heart had a regular rate and rhythm without murmurs. The abdomen was soft without masses, and the extremities were without any bruises, cyanosis, or edema.

Lab Data and Hospital Course: The patient was admitted, and a right anterior nasal pack was placed. Serial hematocrits were also obtained. The night of her first day of admission, she required replacement of an anterior pack because of refractory bleeding. The day following her admission, she was transfused with two units of packed red blood cells for a hemoglobin of 8.

On the second day of her admission, bleeding was noted around the anterior pack. For this reason, she was taken to the treatment room, where a posterior nasopharyngeal pack and a new anterior pack were placed. She was then transferred to the special care unit and monitored on the cardiac monitor and with pulse oximetry. The posterior pack was left in place for two days. At this time, a repeat bleeding showed that her bleeding time had normalized from its previous elevated level. She was observed overnight for one day without any pack in. The patient did well during this observation period without any further bleeding.

When it was confirmed that she had no further bleeding for 48 hours after pack removal, with a stable hematocrit, she was discharged to home. She was instructed to follow up with her private physician. She was also instructed to refrain from taking aspirin and to use Disalcid 750 mg tid, instead, for her arthritic pain. She was also placed on iron supplements 300 mg three times a day and told to continue taking saline and Prenaris nasal drops.

Final Diagnosis: Epistaxis

Additional Diagnosis: Rheumatoid arthritis

1. PDX:

2. Other diagnoses:

3. Principal procedure:

4. Other procedures:

5. Conditions to clarify with physician:

Exercise 2

History of Present Illness: The patient is an 80-year-old white female with a known history of advanced metastatic carcinoma of the breast, widely metastatic. The patient was admitted because of increasing shortness of breath and severe pain. The pain, which was worse in her left chest, was associated with increasing shortness of breath. At the time of admission, the patient was in so much pain she was unable to remember her history. The patient initially presented for congestive heart failure over a year ago. This was subsequently found to be secondary to metastatic breast cancer, post left mastectomy, three years ago. The patient has previously been on chemotherapy.

Lab Data and Hospital Course: The patient was treated initially with IV pain medication to control her pain. Subsequently, she stabilized on oral medication. By the time of discharge, the patient was stable on oral Vicodin and she was able to eat. Blood sugars were improved and her Tolinase was able to be held. Lab at time of discharge included BUN 17, creatinine 1, sodium 141, potassium 4.5, chloride 105, CO_2 25, alkaline phosphatase elevated at 170 with GGT 267, SGOT 68. Admission BUN was up to 38 with creatinine 1.3 secondary to dehydration. By the time of discharge, these had improved. Admission glucose 225, down to 110 at discharge.

Medications at discharge include: Aldactone, 25 mg twice a day; Tamoxifen, 10 mg bid with meals; Lanoxin, 0.125 mg daily; Metamucil, 5 cc in four ounces of juice twice a day; Tolinase, 250 mg half tablet bid (but hold if preceding AccuCheck is less than 125); Reglan, 10 mg po ac; Timoptic 0.5% eye drops, 1 to each eye twice a day; Pepcid, 20 mg bid; Lasix, 40 mg daily (only if pedal edema is present); Vicodin tablets, 1 every three hours prn for pain.

Discharge Diagnosis: Uncontrolled pain, secondary to widely metastatic breast carcinoma. Dehydration. Type II diabetes mellitus, uncontrolled. Congestive heart failure.

1. PDX:

2. Other diagnoses:

3. Principal procedure:

4. Other procedures:

5. Conditions to clarify with physician:

Exercise 3

History of Present Illness: This 70-year-old female with a past history of endometrial carcinoma was admitted to medical oncology for blood transfusion. The patient complains of GI bleeding on and off for the past two months. No changes in bowel movements, no diarrhea, no constipation. There is mild abdominal pain in lower part of abdomen, no radiation, relieved by analgesics. No nausea, no vomiting. Endometrial carcinoma, stage 2, diagnosed in November of last year. Status post radiation therapy externally and internally in January. CT scan of the abdomen in March showed decrease in the size of the mass, and the patient had total abdominal hysterectomy and bilateral salpingo-oophorectomy at that time. The patient presented one month ago with GI bleeding, which was thought to be secondary to radiation colitis, but proctoscopy revealed necrotic mass in anterior wall. Biopsy was negative times two. There is history of hypertension for six years. History of type II diabetes mellitus for 10 years. Medication: Nifedipine, 90 XL once a day; Tolbutamide, 500 mg once a day. No alcohol. Patient smokes one pack of cigarettes per day.

Physical Examination: Alert and oriented in no active distress. Blood pressure 110/60. HEENT: pale conjunctiva. Neck supple, no lymphadenopathy. The lungs were clear to auscultation, resonant to percussion. Heart regular rate and rhythm, no murmurs, no S3. Abdomen soft; there is tenderness in the lower parts; no hepatosplenomegaly. The bowel sounds are positive. Rectal positive for heme. Extremities plus two edema in the left more than the right.

Lab Data: Hemoglobin 6.7, hematocrit 20.8, white blood cells 9.7, neutrophils 81, lymphocytes 14 and monocytes 4, eosinophils 1. Platelet count 448,000. Sodium 142, potassium 4.8, chloride 108, CO_2 21, BUN 40, calcium 8.2, phosphorus 3, magnesium 1.4 and glucose 123, SGOT 50, alkaline phosphatase 137, SGPT 42, albumin 2.0; total bilirubin .3, direct bilirubin 0. PT 11.7, PTT 27.6.

Hospital Course: Problem #1: Lower GI bleed and melena. The patient presented two months ago with lower GI bleed, which was most likely secondary to radiation therapy. At that time, proctoscopy was done and showed necrotic mass in the anterior wall of the rectum. Biopsy was also done and was negative. Proctoscopy was repeated and was negative the second time. For current admission, the patient presented with the same complaint. Hemoglobin was 6.7; hematocrit was 20. The patient was transfused with 4 units of packed red blood. Hemoglobin came up to 14.2, hematocrit to 41.8, and the patient was stabilized. GI people were contacted regarding repeating proctoscopy. Their suggestion was to discharge and follow her in GI clinic.

Problem #2: Endometrial carcinoma, status post radiation therapy, status post resection. No further therapy now.

Problem #3: Anemia, secondary to lower GI bleed.

Problem #4: Type II diabetes mellitus, which is stable on Tolbutamide, 500 mg once a day.

Problem #5: Hypertension, which is stable on Nifedipine, 90 XL once a day.

Problem #6: Increased creatinine and BUN, which was not corrected after the hydration. On discharge, creatinine was 3.2 and BUN was 39. Testing will be repeated as an outpatient. The patient is known to have increased creatinine and BUN, most likely secondary to hypertension. The patient was discharged home in stable condition to be followed up in Oncology. Discharge medications: Nifedipine, 90 XL once a day; Tolbutamide, 500 mg once a day.

Final Diagnosis: Lower gastrointestinal bleeding secondary to radiation colitis.

1. PDX:

2. Other diagnoses:

3. Principal procedure:

4. Other procedures:

5. Conditions to clarify with physician:

Exercise 4

History of Present Illness: The patient is a 72-year-old male who was involved in an interpersonal altercation at approximately 1:30 in the morning. He presented to the emergency department with complaints of pain and swelling to the right side of the face. The patient had been struck multiple times with the butt end of a handgun. He denied loss of consciousness. The attack was witnessed, and the witnesses also claim there was no loss of consciousness. He presented with pain and swelling on the right side of his face in the temporal region and in the right eye region. He had a small abrasion on the top of his head and on the right forehead. No lacerations were noted. He had no diplopia. The past medical and surgical histories were noncontributory. The patient was taking no medications and had no allergies.

Lab Data: Admission x-rays and CT scan revealed a nondisplaced right zygoma fracture and an orbital floor fracture with slight limitation of his upward gaze on physical examination.

Hospital Course: He was taken to the operating room for open reduction of the facial fracture and placement of silastic implant to right orbital floor fracture, which was accomplished without difficulty or complication. The patient tolerated the procedure well. Postoperative course was uncomplicated. He received IV antibiotics throughout his stay in the hospital. Currently, he is tolerating a general diet without problems. He was up and about, ambulating without difficulty. He will be seen here at the hospital on Saturday for suture removal. Discharge medications: Keflex, 500 mg to be taken qid for one week.

Final Diagnoses: Right orbital fracture

Right zygoma fracture

Abrasions of head

Operations: Exploration and placement of silastic implant to right orbital floor fracture

1. PDX: *802.6, 802.4*

2. Other diagnoses: *910.0, E 968.2*

3. Principal procedure: *76.79*

4. Other procedures: *76.92*

5. Conditions to clarify with physician: *IV Antibiotics to what*

Exercise 5

History of Present Illness: This 66-year-old woman was initially admitted on September 1, following a seven-month history of left upper quadrant and left flank abdominal pain. This pain was severe, constant, and not related to food intake. The patient had undergone further workup at her home in Michigan. At that time, only gastritis was found with esophagogastroduodenoscopy and upper gastrointestinal swallow. Thus, the patient chose to come here for further evaluation.

She was admitted on September 1, discharged on September 6, and underwent several diagnostic studies. An ultrasound of the abdomen did not show any evidence of retained gallstones or common duct stones, as she had undergone a cholecystectomy in the past. The patient underwent a computerized tomography scan of her abdomen. The tomography demonstrated a mass in the tail and the body of her pancreas that involved the left kidney and the spleen. There was a question that there was enlarged periaortic nodes and also an enlarged left adrenal gland. The patient also underwent an intravenous pyelogram, which demonstrated splaying of the left kidney. Renal scan demonstrated good renal perfusion to both kidneys. Upper and lower GI endoscopies in this initial hospitalization demonstrated no involvement of the stomach, esophagus, or duodenum, or of the colon.

Because of the severity of the pain, the assessment was that the patient probably had pancreatic carcinoma. Consults were made with the radiology department and the urology service. The final consensus was that this was most likely a pancreatic tumor. The patient had severe, unrelenting pain that was only controlled with narcotics at this time. After a thorough discussion with the patient of the possible treatments, the patient chose to pursue a possible operative resection. The patient stated that the pain appeared to be getting worse and she also was undergoing weight loss. Therefore, the patient was admitted to the hospital.

Hospital Course: The indications for operation in this patient were a possible resection of this tumor for palliation and control of her pain. Based on her computerized tomography scan, it did not appear that this tumor was involved with any other vascular structures that would preclude resection.

On September 12, the patient went to the operating room for left nephrectomy. At this time, she had resection of her distal pancreas and spleen after a left kidney en bloc. However, this tumor involved her celiac access. An operative injury to the superior mesenteric artery was repaired at the time of the operation with a reversed interposition vein graft. Her operative course was complicated by diffuse intravascular coagulation, persistent bleeding, and hypothermia following anesthesia, requiring massive blood transfusions. Following revascularization of her small bowel, the patient needed to be packed and was returned to the surgical intensive care unit in critical condition.

The patient had a rocky postoperative course and arrested several times in the first four hours following return to the intensive care unit. Four hours following her return to the intensive care unit, the patient arrested and could not be resuscitated. The final cause of death was carcinoma of the pancreas and was related to resection of this cancer.

Final Diagnosis: Carcinoma of the tail of the pancreas with extension to spleen and left kidney

1. PDX: *157.2*
2. Other diagnoses: *197.4, 198.0, 998.2, 902.25, 995.89, 427.5, 998.11* *286.6*
3. Principal procedure: *52.52*
4. Other procedures: *41.5, 55.51, 39.56 88.01*
5. Conditions to clarify with physician:

Exercise 6

History of Present Illness: This 87-year-old female is a known type II diabetic who underwent an amputation of her fourth digit of the right foot approximately five weeks ago. She was referred elsewhere for angioplasty. At that time, she was taken off her insulin and is currently being treated with a 1,500-calorie diabetic diet. She was sent back to the nursing home and has since developed an increasing amount of pain and cellulitis of her right foot. The patient is a poor historian. She is alert, but her orientation seems to be off. Information is obtained from her old records and from the transfer sheet sent from the nursing home. Feb. 2004: pacemaker implantation secondary to sick sinus syndrome with congestive heart failure (stable with Lasix, 40 mg po) and bradyarrhythmia, as well as pleural effusion. Oct. 2006: acute MI.

Physical Examination: General: Reveals an 87-year-old white female in no acute distress. BP 152/70, temperature 99.8 orally, pulse 66, respirations 24. Skin: Warm and dry. HEENT: Head is normocephalic, atraumatic. Pupils are equal, round, and reactive to light and accommodation. Extraocular muscles are intact. Fundi are not visualized. No conjunctivitis or icterus noted. Canals are clear with good cone of light reflex on TMs. Gross hearing is within normal limits. Septum is midline. No discharge. No erythema or exudate of throat. Uvula raises midline. Neck: Supple with full range of motion. No lymphadenopathy or thyromegaly. No carotid bruits or JVD. Breasts: No masses or nipple discharge. Lungs: Clear on the left with rales in right lower lobe. Heart: Grade II/VI systolic ejection murmur elicited with a paced beat. Abdomen: Distended. Positive bowel sounds X4. No hepatosplenomegaly. No masses upon palpation. GU: Rectal: Deferred at this time. Musculoskeletal: Right foot is status post fourth toe amputation with open incision with exudate, as well as surrounding erythema of approximately 3 cm. Skin is warm to touch and tender. Right arm paralysis with slight weakness of the right leg. Neuro: Cranial nerves II through XII grossly intact. No major deficits noted.

Impression: Cellulitis of right foot, s/p amputation; non-insulin-dependent diabetes mellitus; arteriosclerotic heart disease with history of sick sinus syndrome and pacemaker implantation; and residual right hemiparesis from cerebral thrombosis.

Plan: Admit for IV antibiotics.

Hospital Course: Following angioplasty, it was thought the circulation was good in her foot at the time of her discharge from St. Mary's Hospital. However, soon after returning to the nursing home, she began having increasing cellulitis, which led to her being brought here. Culture revealed a Staph aureus. Admission white count was essentially normal with 7,800 white cells, 80 Segs. Glucose was 149 with normal follow-up. Urinalysis was normal. Creatinine was 1.5; BUN was 18; platelet count was normal. Dig. level was high normal. The patient was treated with bed rest, elevation of the foot, Betadine soaks, IV Garamycin, and Cleocin. With the treatment here, the patient's pain subsided. Doppler pressures in her ankle were adequate. The wound drainage became much less. At the time of her discharge to Skilled Care, there was no real evidence of cellulitis. However, I think she will benefit from continued intravenous antibiotic therapy and local care. She was discharged to Skilled Care to continue the intravenous Garamycin and Cleocin.

Diagnoses: Cellulitis, right foot, post amputation

Diabetes mellitus

Diabetic peripheral vascular disease with recent angioplasty

1. PDX:

2. Other diagnoses:

3. Principal procedure:

4. Other procedures:

5. Conditions to clarify with physician:

Exercise 7

History of Present Illness: This is a 69-year-old female with previous MI, known hypertensive, who started complaining of cough, chills, and fever about 4 days prior to admission. One day prior to admission, she started to complain of progressive dyspnea associated with hemoptysis. She went to the emergency department and was noted to be extremely dyspneic and wheezing. She was given an aerosol treatment with good response. However, chest x-ray showed evidence of bilateral lower pneumonia with a PO_2 of 66 and white blood cell count of 12,400, for which admission was advised. The patient had been taking Methyldopa 500 mg bid, Ascriptin 1 tablet daily, Transderm Nitro 5 once daily, Capoten 30 mg bid, and Lanoxin .725 mg daily. The patient had an inferior wall myocardial infarction 10 months ago. She is known to have chronic anxiety problems and had been under the care of the Mental Hygiene Clinic.

Physical Examination: Revealed a well-developed, well-nourished female whose respirations had improved since the aerosol therapy was given. Blood pressure is somewhat elevated. Respirations 24. Pulse 110/minute. HEENT: Unremarkable. No carotid bruits. No distended neck veins. Chest: No deformity. Equal expansion. Lungs: Crepitant rales over the lower half of end hemithorax. No wheezing. No pericardial or pleural rub noted. Heart: Regular rhythm. No murmurs. Abdomen: Soft. Liver, spleen, and kidneys not enlarged. No tenderness. Extremities: No clubbing. No cyanosis. Peripheral pulses strong and equal. Rectal: Deferred.

Impression: Lobar pneumonia associated with hemoptysis. Previous inferior wall myocardial infarction. Hypertension. Chronic anxiety.

Plan: After appropriate cultures are obtained, the patient will be empirically started on Kefzol. Nasal oxygen will be administered. Patient will be hydrated and aerosol therapy will be continued.

Lab Data and Hospital Course: Sputum smear showed moderate white blood cells, many epithelial cells, and many mixed respiratory microflora. Sputum culture showed normal growth. Blood cultures after 10 days showed no growth. Chest x-ray report revealed mild congestive cardiac failure pattern. Significant improvement in congestive heart failure noted on second x-ray, but not complete resolution, although the pneumonia has resolved. EKG showed right bundle branch block with old inferior myocardial infarction, left ventricular strain; no change when this was repeated prior to discharge. The patient's previous medications were continued.

After cultures were obtained, she was empirically started on IV Kefzol. Because of initial bronchospasm, she was also started on aerosolized bronchodilator therapy consisting of Alupent. She remained afebrile during her stay in the hospital. She had no further wheezing after 24 hours, but continued to have mild hemoptysis and crepitant rales in both bases. Hemoptysis disappeared after 48 hours. She had one episode of mild angina pains relieved by nitroglycerin during her stay. With improvement in her respirations and x-ray findings, she was discharged. Her BP was 154/110 on discharge, but this is not considered unusual since her BP is quite unstable as an outpatient, with variable high and low readings. This will, however, be followed up in the office.

Final Diagnoses: Bilateral lobar pneumonia and hemoptysis

Old myocardial infarction with angina

Hypertension

Chronic anxiety

Congestive heart failure

1. PDX:

2. Other diagnoses:

3. Principal procedure:

4. Other procedures:

5. Conditions to clarify with physician:

Exercise 8

History of Present Illness: The patient is a 72-year-old male with a history of abdominal perineal resection for colon cancer in 1994 and left hemicolectomy in 1995 for splenic flexure recurrence of cancer. Subsequent right nephrectomy, right adrenalectomy, right posterior hepatic wedge resection in February for metastatic colon carcinoma. The patient is admitted with complaints of lower back pain and bilateral thigh pain times two months, increasing in intensity.

Physical Examination: Examination on admission: temperature 99, pulse 72, respirations 24, blood pressure 150/90. The examination was remarkable for left lower quadrant colostomy from previous operation, mildly tender lumbar spine, and the patient was barely able to stand. It was also noted that the patient had decreased sharp, dull discrimination on the neural examination of the lateral thighs.

Lab Data: On admission the labs were: Urinalysis: specific gravity 1.021, pH 5; Chem tests were negative; Nitrite negative; Blood negative, 12 white cells, moderate bacteria. The clinical chemistry results were: serum sodium 141, BUN 42, potassium 4.9, chloride 104, CO_2 28, glucose 99, creatinine 1.8, SGOT 12, SGPT 16, alkaline phosphatase 68, total protein 6.6, albumin 3.8, total bilirubin 0.7, direct bilirubin 0.0, GGT 87, calcium 10.3, magnesium 2.0, phosphorus 3.2, uric acid 5.7, PT 12.9, PTT 28.4, white count 8.0, hemoglobin 15.0, hematocrit 43.8, platelets 223,000. The CEA level was noted to be 508 nanograms per mL on admission. Metastatic workup for the colon carcinoma revealed no evidence of metastatic disease to the head or the thoracic and cervical spine.

Radiologic Studies: CT and MRI revealed left celiac ganglion node plexus enlarged, suspicious for metastasis. Multiple small lung nodules bilaterally suspicious for metastasis. Pathological fracture of L2, with compression of L2, effacement of the spinal canal space and apparent cord compression at the L2 level. Subsequent urine culture grew out greater than 10 to the 5th pseudomonas aeruginosa, which was sensitive to Ciprofloxacin. The patient was treated with Ciprofloxacin 500 mg po q eight hours and subsequent urine culture showed no growth.

Hospital Course: The patient went to the operating room for L-2 laminectomy with decompression and anterior allograft bone fusion. The postoperative course was marked by slow recovery with nausea and difficulty with pain control. The patient slowly improved and began ambulating eight days later. The patient fell three days later on ambulation but was without significant injuries. Further physical therapy was marked by continued improvement in ambulation with walker and no further setbacks. Clinically, the patient is afebrile without signs and symptoms of infection, no CVA tenderness, no dysuria. The patient will be discharged home today. Condition on discharge fairly good.

Treatment: The patient will go home on Vicodin po q 4–6 hours for pain and Capoten. He will resume Capoten bid dosing per his internist's recommendations, 25 po bid. Prognosis: The long-term prognosis is poor as the patient has metastatic colon CA; short-term prognosis is fairly good with improvement in ambulation. Ambulation with assistance with walker. Follow-up: The patient will return to see me next Wednesday.

Final Diagnoses: Metastatic colon cancer to lung and bone

Pathologic compression fracture of L2 vertebra with cord compression at L2 level

UTI due to Pseudomonas

1.   PDX:

2.   Other diagnoses:

3.   Principal procedure:

4.   Other procedures:

5.   Conditions to clarify with physician:

Exercise 9

History of Present Illness: This 71-year-old male was the pedestrian in a pedestrian versus motor vehicle accident. He had no loss of consciousness at the scene but was confused at the time of admission. He had vital signs that were stable in the field. He sustained head lacerations.

Physical Examination: The patient was alert, but confused. He was in a cervical collar and had a laceration of the scalp posteriorly and a small laceration under the chin. Chest: Clear to auscultation. Heart: Regular. Abdomen: Soft and nontender with positive bowel sounds. He had a palpable right inguinal hernia, which was large. Extremities: His pedal pulses were intact bilaterally. He was able to move all extremities well. Head and neck examination: Revealed eyes intact. Neck was nontender to palpation, but the patient remained in the C-collar.

Lab Data and Hospital Course: Chest x-ray and EKG revealed no gross lesions. The EKG revealed atrial fibrillation. Laboratory examination was unremarkable. Chest x-ray revealed cardiomegaly. Odontoid tomograms did not show a fracture. He had a right small subarachnoid hemorrhage on his head CT scan. The patient was admitted to the Intensive Care Unit for observation. He was stable in the Intensive Care Unit and was transferred to the ward, where he was monitored on telemetry. Social Work was immediately contacted for discharge planning. Neurosurgery was consulted. They felt the patient had a traumatic subarachnoid hemorrhage, which was small, and they would follow it clinically. They stated that he had a history of syncope and suggested an MRI of his head.

On February 7, the patient was attempting to ambulate when the Trauma Service noted he had left knee pain. Radiographs revealed a Schatzker IV tibial plateau fracture. The patient was then evaluated preoperatively for open reduction internal fixation of his left lower extremity. Preoperative laboratories were unremarkable. Both the patient and his wife then refused surgery. It was then opted to treat the tibial plateau fracture in a long-leg plaster cast. Radiographs following placement of the plaster showed adequate reduction of the fracture. It was discussed with the patient and his wife that the patient may require arthroplasty of the knee in the future, but that the tibial fracture would be well treated in the plaster. It was the preference of the operative team to perform open reduction internal fixation, but the patient and his wife were against an operative procedure at that time. Psychiatry was also consulted to evaluate the competency of the patient. They felt that the patient was somewhat demented, but that he did understand the benefits and risks of surgery and was competent to make decisions.

On 2/9, the patient was noted to be quite lethargic and had apnea as well. Neurosurgery evaluated the patient and administered IV fluids. They checked laboratories and found the patient was hypovolemic. The patient improved following administration of IV fluids. By 2/10, the patient was oriented and much improved. He was discharged to home on 2/15. At the time of discharge, vital signs were stable and he was afebrile. Circulation, motor, and sensory were intact to his left lower extremity. The plaster was intact.

Final Diagnoses: Closed head trauma with subarachnoid hemorrhage

Closed left tibial plateau fracture

Dementia senile

Hypovolemia

1. PDX:

2. Other diagnoses:

3. Principal procedure:

4. Other procedures:

5. Conditions to clarify with physician:

Exercise 10

History of Present Illness: The patient is a 75-year-old female with coronary arteriosclerosis status post coronary artery bypass graft. The patient presents complaining of shortness of breath that began three to four days prior to admission and became worse on the day of admission. She complains of wheezing and cough productive of whitish sputum. No fever, chills, nausea, or vomiting. Paroxysmal nocturnal dyspnea, orthopnea is unchanged. Past medical history, as above.

Physical Examination: On physical examination, the patient is alert and oriented, in mild distress. Her blood pressure is 150/70, heart rate 70, respiratory rate 16. The temperature is afebrile. The head and neck examinations are within normal limits. Patient wheezes. Abdomen soft, nontender. The extremities are 2+ edema bilaterally. Neurological: Left upper extremity and left lower extremities were weak and unable to ambulate.

Lab Data: The WBC is 7.5, hemoglobin 11.0, hematocrit 34.2. The platelets are 292,000. The Digoxin level is 0.5. The chest x-ray revealed cardiomegaly and congestive heart failure. Pulmonary vascularity within normal limits. The sodium is 143, potassium 4.5, chloride 111, bicarbonate 21. The BUN is 23, creatinine 1.2, glucose 207.

Hospital Course: The patient was admitted with chronic obstructive pulmonary disease exacerbation. She responded well to nebulized breathing treatments and intravenous Solu-Medrol. She was then switched to po steroids. The patient was discharged home in stable condition on the following medications: Prednisone 40 mg on an untapering dose; aspirin, enteric-coated, one po q am; Atrovent and albuterol inhaler; Persantine 75 mg tid; Captopril 12.5 mg tid; Theophylline 300 mg bid; Diltiazem 90 mg tid; Nitropaste 7.5 mg q am; Lasix 40 mg q am; and Digoxin .25 mg q am. She is to follow up in two weeks in the Pulmonary Clinic. The patient also has follow-up in the Cardiology Clinic.

Final Diagnosis: Acute exacerbation of chronic obstructive pulmonary disease

Secondary Diagnoses: Congestive heart failure, acute diastolic

Diabetes mellitus type II controlled by diet

Hypertension

1.   PDX:

2.   Other diagnoses:

3.   Principal procedure:

4.   Other procedures:

5.   Conditions to clarify with physician:

Case Studies

Directions

Under the inpatient prospective payment system (IPPS), health record documentation must support the principal diagnosis and principal procedure, as well as all other diagnoses and procedures submitted on the claim.

The coder should review the documentation to identify:

1. The principal diagnosis, which may not be the diagnosis listed first by the physician

2. The principal procedure

3. Other diagnoses and procedures to be included on the claim

4. Any other diagnoses or procedures that require coding for the healthcare facility to have appropriate databases

In selecting diagnoses/procedures for coding, the coder should assume that the documentation provided is the only documentation available. If no documentation is available to indicate that a condition affected treatment or length of stay, do not code this condition. Identify these types of conditions on the answer sheet in the space titled "Issues to clarify with physician."

On the job, the coder may review other sections of the health record and consult with the attending physician, if necessary, for assistance in sequencing and code selection. In the following cases, however, the information available to the coder is limited. Answers for each sequencing/coding scenario must be based solely on sequencing guidelines, ICD-9-CM coding conventions and principles, the PPS regulations, and the information provided in the case.

Case 1

History

Chief Complaint: Feeling weak and passing bright red blood

History of Present Illness: The patient says for the last three days he has had huge amounts of bright red blood going through his rectum. Yesterday, this seemed to slow down; he just had a little black color on top of the stool, but there was no bright red blood. He denies any abdominal pain, fever, chills, or back pain. No nausea or vomiting. No runny nose or cough. He says most of the blood was in the toilet bowl and some was on the tissue paper. This a.m., he had a little bit of nausea while eating lunch. He also is complaining of some chest pain, which was dull and lasted for about 1½ hours after he ate lunch. This was not like his previous MI pain. He denies any diaphoresis.

I saw him in the office on Feb. 11, with all his symptoms. I did an EKG in the office and it did not show any change. He looked a little bit pale. I scheduled him for a flexible sigmoidoscopy and did a CBC. The CBC came back later on the same day saying the hematocrit was about 22. I did a flexible sigmoidoscopy on him after admission this morning. The bowel prep was inadequate. Almost all the sigmoid colon was covered with loose, slightly greenish stool, but a whole lot of diverticula was all over the sigmoid colon. I could go up to 45 cm, but there was a lot more stool and I could not get past it. The patient was also complaining of pain, so I stopped the sigmoidoscopy at that time. The patient also states he has been feeling pretty weak. He denies any shortness of breath, paroxysmal nocturnal dyspnea, or swelling of the feet.

Past Medical History: Significant for: (1) Chronic back pain. He is status post laminectomy of L5-S1 five years ago. He recently had some surgery in the lower back and also some surgery in the cervical spine with stenosis. (2) He had degenerative joint disease. (3) He says he had an MI about 20 or 25 years ago. (4) History of hypercholesterolemia. (5) Status post carotid endarterectomy about 5 or 8 years ago. (6) History of CVA with right hemiparesis, more than 5 years ago; complete recovery. (7) Extreme anxiety. (8) He does exhibit some sleeping pill addictive behavior. He has been weaned off a lot of sleeping pills. He used to take Valium (up to 50 mg) in the past. He was also taking a lot of Percocet for his back pain. He is off all those medications. The only medication he takes is Restoril, 15–20 mg at bedtime.

Family History: Mother died with stomach cancer. Father had angina, no MI.

Social History: He used to be in the dry-cleaning business. He does not smoke now and quit smoking 20 years ago. No alcohol. He lives with his wife at home.

Review of Systems: As per HPI and PMH.

Physical Examination

The patient is alert and in no distress, somewhat pale.

Neck: Supple. No JVD. Good carotid upstrokes.

Lungs: Clear.

Heart: S1 and S2. Grade I over VI systolic murmur.

Abdomen: Soft, nontender. No masses are felt. No hepatosplenomegaly. Bowel sounds are normal. There is no pedal edema.

Rectal: Definitely heme positive.

Impression: Patient is a 74-year-old white male with lower GI bleed and anemia, probably secondary to the lower GI bleed. He is symptomatic with anemia. Will admit him to the hospital and give him blood. Will get a barium enema tomorrow to see if there is any etiology of his lower GI bleed other than diverticula, which are probably bleeding. He has had one such episode in the past. We want to make sure he has no evidence of any carcinoma or any other etiology for cancer while he is here in the hospital.

Progress Notes

2/13   Doing fine. Hemoccult neg. Lungs clear. Hct about 27 today.

2/14   Hemoccult neg. No major complaints. Says he is feeling much stronger.
        Exam: WNL
        Hgb/Hct: 9.2/28.4
        B.E shows extensive diverticula

Discharge Dx: Blood loss anemia secondary to bleeding diverticula, anxiety
                     D/C home on FeSO4 and lots of fiber
                     F/U in 3–5 days

Radiology Consultation

Barium Enema: Examination of the colon with barium shows no constant filling defect or mucosal ulceration. There are multiple, somewhat large diverticula involving the left colon. No extrinsic pressure deformity is noted. Scattered loops of small bowel are noted without evidence of reflux into the terminal ileum.

Impression: Rather marked diverticulosis of the left colon without evidence of diverticulitis. Suggestion of some small bowel ileus.

Laboratory Tests

Test	2/12	2/13	2/14	Reference	Units
WBC	6.2		5.7	4.8–10.8	x10-3
RBC	3.06 L		3.93 L	4.70–6.10	x10-6
Hemoglobin	6.4 C (1)	8.9 C	(*) 9.2 L	14.0–18.0	9
Hematocrit	20.8 C (1)	27.8 L	(*) 28.4	42.0–52.0	%
MCV	67.9 L		72.3 L	80.0–94.0	u3
MCH	20.9 L		23.4 L	27.0–31.0	uug
MCHC	30.8 L		32.4	32.0–36.0	%
RDW	17.6 H		20.3 H	11.8–14.1	%
Platelet Estimate	Adequate		Adequate	Adequate	
SEGS	67		71H	40–70	%
Bands	0		0	0–4	%
Eosinophils	0		1	0–3	%
Basophils	1		0	0–1	%
Lymphocytes	30		25	20–45	%
Monocytes	2		3	0–4	%
Metamyelocytes	0		0	0–0	%
Myelocytes	0		0	0–0	%
Anisocytosis	2+ A		3+ A		
Poikilocytosis	1+ A		1+ A		
Microcytic			1+ A		
Hypochromia	3+ A		1+ A		
Polychromia			1+ A		
Test Result Comments					
*1 Result verified by repeat analysis					

Transfusion Service   **Product Chart Copy**

Patient Data   Blood Product

PATIENT ID: 55951   MR/ACCT #: 2177186   UNIT #: 16T69389

NAME: COMPONENT: PRC Packed Red Cells

LOCATION: 2N   ABO/Rh: 0 POS   ABO/Rh: 0 POS
   2 North

SPECIAL NEEDS: REMARKS:

SEX: M   BIRTHDATE: 08/02/1917

Crossmatch Compatible? YES   Crossmatch Date/Time: 02/12 13:35

Specimen In-Date/Time: 02/12 12:05 Tech:

Antibody Screen: NEG

Transfusion Service Comments:

Need where?:   When?:   Ordering Physician:

Nursing Unit Instructions: Blood Warmer Temp: C

I have checked this slip with bag labels and the Patient wristband and started the
transfusion:

NAME _____ RN MD TRANSFUSION STARTED: _____ _____
                                                        (date)   (time)

PRETRANSFUSION VITAL SIGNS: Blood Pressure   Pulse   Temperature
POST TRANSFUSION VITAL SIGNS: Blood Pressure   Pulse   Temperature
TRANSFUSION COMPLETED: _____   _____am/pm   AMOUNT TRANSFUSED: _____ml
                 (date)   (time)   REACTION NOTED? ___ YES ___ NO

* *
* *

Transfusion Service   **Product Chart Copy**

Patient Data   Blood Product

PATIENT ID: 55951   MR/ACCT #: 2177186   UNIT #: 16T69389

NAME: COMPONENT: PRC Packed Red Cells

LOCATION: 2N   ABO/Rh: 0 POS   ABO/Rh: 0 POS
   2 North

SPECIAL NEEDS: REMARKS:

SEX: M   BIRTHDATE: 08/02/1917

Crossmatch Compatible?: YES   Crossmatch Date/Time: 02/12 13:35

Specimen In-Date/Time: 02/12 12:05 Tech:

Antibody Screen: NEG

Transfusion Service Comments:

Need where?   When?   Ordering Physician:

Nursing Unit Instructions: Blood Warmer Temp: C

I have checked this slip with bag labels and the Patient wristband and started the
transfusion:

NAME _____ RN MD TRANSFUSION STARTED: _____ _____
                                                        (date)   (time)

PRETRANSFUSION VITAL SIGNS: Blood Pressure   Pulse   Temperature
POST TRANSFUSION VITAL SIGNS: Blood Pressure   Pulse   Temperature
TRANSFUSION COMPLETED: _____   _____am/pm   AMOUNT TRANSFUSED: _____ml
                 (date)   (time)   REACTION NOTED? ___ YES ___ NO

Case 1: Solution

1. Principal diagnosis: _____

    _____

2. Other diagnoses: _____

    _____

3. Procedures: _____

    _____

4. Issues to clarify with physician: _____

    _____

Case 2

Discharge Summary

Patient is a 78-year-old female. She saw the doctor recently with abdominal pain and constipation. A barium enema showed diverticulosis and perhaps a stricture near the sigmoid and rectal junction. She was scoped by the doctor, who saw a stricture at that point and said he couldn't rule out a carcinoma. Upper GI showed a hiatal hernia and duodenal diverticulum. Ultrasound showed gallstones. The patient had some bladder incontinence. She has had atrial fibrillation, diabetes, and takes Lanoxin. Otherwise, she is doing quite well. She has had a previous right total hip.

At the time of admission, it was felt that she had a stricture, rule out carcinoma, diabetes mellitus, exogenous obesity, past history of atrial fibrillation, previous abdominal hysterectomy, previous right total hip. Her chest film showed some chronic blunting of the right costophrenic angle, but otherwise was negative. Her admission EKG showed what was thought to be a normal sinus rhythm. Her blood type was AB-Positive. Urinalysis was negative. Hemoglobin was 13.3, white count 7,600. Protime 12, PTT was 23. The CEA, which came back several days later, was quite high at 856. Glucose is 127, albumin is 3.4. Other labs were normal.

After mechanical and chemical bowel prep, she was taken to surgery. First, we laparoscoped her to see if we could do this resection with the scope. When we found that it was adherent to loops of adjacent small bowel, she had an open resection. A large carcinoma of the rectosigmoid junction was found and resected with an end-to-end anastomosis. A segment of small bowel that was stuck to the tumor was also resected, with a functional end-to-end anastomosis done. At least four separate liver metastases were noted. Needle biopsy of that was done as well. The pathology report showed moderate to poorly differentiated carcinoma, bases through the wall of the colon and into the perirectal fat. The small intestine was not involved. The liver metastases were also positive.

The patient had a rather smooth postoperative course. She was thought to be ready for discharge on the sixth post-operative day. She was seen in consultation prior to surgery by the doctor, who managed her medical problems and diabetes and will arrange for appropriate medication at the time of discharge. She was sent home on Darvocet for pain. Ferrous Gluconate 324 mg three times a day for a month to restore her blood count. She is to resume her other previous medications. She is to restrict her activities for two months and to see me in the office in eight days.

Final Diagnosis:

1. Invasive adenocarcinoma of the rectosigmoid, metastatic to the liver
2. Type 2 diabetes mellitus
3. Exogenous obesity
4. Atrial fibrillation
5. Previous right total hip replacement
6. Previous abdominal hysterectomy

Operative Procedure: Resection of rectosigmoid with low pelvic anastomosis with an EEA, small bowel resection, liver biopsy.

History

Patient is a 78-year-old female. She has been in to see the doctor recently with abdominal pain and complains that she was unable to move her bowels. She was admitted and subsequently had endoscopy following a number of x-rays.

The x-rays showed diverticulosis of the sigmoid and perhaps a stricture near the sigmoid rectal junction. This was difficult to delineate because of overlapping loops of bowel. The patient had an upper GI showing hiatal hernia and a duodenal diverticulum, and an ultrasound showing gallstones.

The patient was subsequently seen by the doctor. A week ago today, the doctor performed upper GI endoscopy, which showed a little antral gastritis. A sigmoidoscopic examination showed, at about 25 cm, a narrowed area of the bowel with edema and stricture, and some blood oozing from above. Doctor said that he could not be sure whether this was strictly a diverticular stricture or whether there was a tumor above this point. The patient has otherwise been pretty healthy.

She had a previous hysterectomy. She had a previous fracture in the right hip. She had pulmonary embolus secondary to thrombophlebitis in her legs on 2 different occasions. She is not a smoker and seldom drinks.

She has no known allergies.

She has 3 children. Both parents are deceased.

She has had type II diabetes for about 5 years and takes Tolinase 150 mg two times a day. She has had atrial fibrillation in the past and takes Lanoxin 0.125 mg a day for that condition. She has never had hypertension, heart disease (other than the atrial fibrillation), or stroke. She has no chest pain or shortness of breath.

She has had quite a bit of heartburn and indigestion, but this definitely has been improved by Zantac.

She has some bladder incontinence.

Physical Examination

She weighs 174. She is 5' 6 1/2" tall. BP 152/84 on the right, 148/78 on the left. Pulse was 80.

Examination of the HEENT was negative. The patient seemed extremely alert. She has good carotid pulses without bruits. No goiter or nodes in the neck. Breasts were somewhat pendant, but there were no masses, no skin or nipple retraction, no axillary supraclavicular nodes.

The heart rate was regular. The heart was not enlarged. There was no murmur. The lungs were clear to auscultation and percussion.

There was a low midline scar. No hepatosplenomegaly. There was a little left lower quadrant tenderness.

Rectal and vaginal exams were not repeated.

She had good femoral, popliteal, and dorsalis pedis pulses. The ankles were quite thick. There was a scar on her right hip from previous surgery.

Neurological is normal.

Her skin tended to be sweaty and clammy, which she says is the normal case for her.

Impression:

1. Stricture of the sigmoid seen on barium enema and colonoscopy, probably secondary to diverticular disease, causing obstructive symptoms
2. Type II diabetes mellitus
3. Exogenous obesity
4. Past history of atrial fibrillation, past previous history of abdominal hysterectomy

Plan: Resection.

Consultation

It was a pleasure to see your patient, who is well known to me from my office. She is a pleasant 78-year-old white, obese female who, over the past 3–4 months, has had increasing amounts of difficulty with bowel movements. She has a complaint of small, pencil-thin bowel movements with some blood noted. The patient also had some difficulty with upper GI indigestion, as well as gastritis. She has been evaluated per gastroenterology at the hospital and diagnosed with antral gastritis as well as diverticulosis, diverticulitis with narrowing of the sigmoid colon, approximately 25 cm via colonoscopy. The patient has had a workup that included an upper GI series and endoscopies that have shown the above problem, etiology yet to be determined. The patient has a rather strong family history of having similar type of etiologies. Apparently, her three sisters have had similar surgeries, surgery-like etiology secondary to narrowing of sigmoid colon, and difficulties with irritable bowel–type symptoms. The patient has had difficulty with her bowel movements for many years. However, during the past three months they have become somewhat more bloody, as well as worsened in types. The patient came to my office approximately three months ago with the above etiology. Workup was done then and is on previous chart for review.

Her past medical history is consistent with type II diabetes mellitus. She is currently on Tolinase bid with fairly good control at home when the patient follows her diet. The patient does not have a history of smoking, nor does she drink. She currently lives alone. The patient had a hip replacement approximately a year or year and half ago with no sequelae. The patient has previous history of pulmonary embolus. However, she has had no difficulty with the previous surgery noted.

The medication protocol at home includes one-a-day aspirin and Tolinase bid basis. She is also taking Lanoxin 0.125 mg for previous history of atrial fibrillation, which has currently been controlled with normal sinus rhythm for the last one-year period of time noted.

The patient has been evaluated for urinary incontinence secondary to a low-lying bladder. Surgical history includes a hysterectomy many years ago. The patient has been in fairly good health except for mild diabetes mellitus, which is controlled with diet as well as oral medications. Otherwise, she has done well and has been in fairly stable condition up to the recent history with her colon problems.

On physical examination, the patient's general HEENT, eyes, ears, nose, and throat are basically clear. Neck does not show any cervical nodes. Neck is clear for adenopathy. Lungs are clear to auscultation; no rales, rhonchi, or friction rubs. No wheezing. The heart rate is regular rate and rhythm. Abdomen is soft, not overtly tender at this time. Extremities do not show any edema. Cranial nerves are grossly intact as tested.

The patient's EKG shows that of normal sinus rhythm, as evaluated by the consultant. The lab work shows a glucose of 127. BUN and creatinine are within normal limits, as are the electrolytes. Albumin is slightly low at 3.4, with a total protein of 6.0. The liver function profile, SGOT, alk. phos., and bilirubin are within normal limits, as well as triglycerides.

Diagnostic Impressions:

1. Diverticulosis/diverticulitis with sigmoid constriction, etiology to be determined, rule out primary disease, that of diverticulosis or diverticulitis versus overt tumor

2. Diabetes mellitus

3. Atrial fibrillation by history, current normal sinus rhythm

4. Generalized obesity

Recommendation:

1. Will put the patient on medication protocol, Lanoxin for control of atrial fibrillation, normal sinus rhythm.

2. Will start a sliding scale Insulin, with regular Humulin Insulin while she is undergoing surgery. Back on Tolinase postsurgery if control is indicated at that time.

Operative Record

Preoperative Diagnosis: Probable diverticular stricture of the sigmoid, rule out carcinoma

Postoperative Diagnosis: Carcinoma of the sigmoid invading into adjacent small bowel with metastases to the liver

Procedure: Attempted laparoscopic bowel removal, open exploration with resection of the sigmoid colon and end-to-end anastomosis with 28 mm EEA. Resection of segment of small bowel with direct extension of the tumor into that area with the functional end-to-end anastomosis, doing a side-to-side anastomosis, biopsy of liver metastases.

Patient is a 78-year-old female who presented with abdominal pain and constipation. Barium enema suggested diverticular stricture. Patient was seen in consultation by the doctor, who sigmoidoscoped the patient and found a stricture at about 25 cm. Doctor could not see above the stricture, so we could not rule out carcinoma. Patient understood the nature of the problem, the proposed operative risk, and its possible complications, and consented to it. She was given a mechanical and chemical bowel prep.

Patient was brought to surgery and an NG tube was placed in the stomach and a Foley in the bladder. She was placed in the lithotomy position, routine prep and drape were done. We made a small incision in the right upper quadrant, directly into the peritoneal cavity and inserted the Hasson cannula, insufflated the peritoneal cavity with CO_2. Once we had a good tent, we examined the peritoneal cavity and could not really see the liver because we were so close to it. We then dissected out the sigmoid after we put in three other cannulas, a 12-mm in the right lower quadrant, a 10-mm in the left lower quadrant, and a 5-mm in the left upper quadrant. These were put in under direct vision. We then grasped the sigmoid and dissected it off the left pelvic gutter, and dissected down toward the bladder. She had undergone a previous hysterectomy, but there were no anterior adhesions. We could not get the small bowel to easily come up out of the pelvis. We then put the colonoscope through the rectum and came up to 25 cm, where we saw not a diverticular stricture, but a carcinoma. We marked this point.

When we were dissecting, we found the small bowel to be adherent at this time and we elected to open, so the trocars and instruments were all removed. We then made a midline incision and, on inspection, found a large mass in the pelvis. We had already freed up the left side of the sigmoid colon with laparoscope. We identified the ureter and pushed it away, opened the right pelvic peritoneum and identified the right ureter, and then transected the bowel above the junction of the sigmoid and descending colon with the GIA. We then divided the mesentery between Kelly clamps, including the inferior mesenteric terminal branch. These were all divided and ligated with heavy silks. We pulled the small bowel off the side, but it did look like there was some direct invasion there, and then further mobilized the tumor and the upper rectum. We divided all the mesentery between Kelly clamps and ligated with heavy silk. We then transected the rectum through its middle and upper one thirds, with TA55 on the distal side and Kocher on the proximal side, and then removed the specimen. We brought the proximal end of the bowel out, cleaned it off of fat and mesentery, put a pursestring instrument on it, excised the bowel distal to the pursestring instrument, opened the pursestring instrument, and then incised it. The size was 28mm. We then put the anvil of EEA in the proximal bowel and tightened it down with pursestring. We put the EEA instrument up through the rectum, pushed the trocar up through the suture line, then connected the anvil to the EEA instrument and tightened it down under direct vision, cut the bowel making the anastomosis and removed the EEA. We then filled the pelvis with saline, clamped the bowel proximally, and put in the colonoscope to obtain a good anastomosis with no bleeding and no leak of air.

We then aspirated the fluid in the pelvis. We resected the segment of the small bowel with GIA and did a functional end-to-end anastomosis and transected the bowel loop outside the anastomosis with a TA55. We actually had done this before we completed the rectal anastomosis, and when we went back we found a hematoma in the mesentery. We dissected through the hematoma to get it controlled, ligated the bleeders with heavy silk, but then we had to resect another 10 cm of small bowel and then did another functional end-to-end anastomosis and closed the enterotomy with TA55 and the mesentery with fine silks. This gave us a nice anastomosis with good pink bowel, pretty close to the cecum.

We then noted there to be at least three, maybe four, metastases scattered over different areas of the right lobe of the liver. One was biopsied with a Tru-cut needle and the biopsy site cauterized. We then had a correct sponge, instrument, and needle count. We closed the fascia of the right upper quadrant puncture wound with some interrupted silk Vicryls and closed the muscles with interrupted Vicryls. The other smaller ports were closed by skin clips. We then closed the fascia of the peritoneum of the midline wound with running suture of #I Vicryl and the fascia with interrupted figure 8 #I Vicryl, closed the skin with clips, and applied sterile dressings. Sponge, instruments, and sharp counts were again correct. The patient tolerated the procedure well and we trust she will do well.

Pathology Report

Specimen-Origin:

I.   Small bowel sigmoid colon

II. Liver biopsy

Pathologic Diagnosis:

I.   Segments of small bowel: Serosal adhesions

Colon: Invasive adenocarcinoma, moderate to poorly differentiated, extending into pericolic adipose

Lymph nodes, small bowel mesentery: Negative for metastasis (0/6 nodes)

Lymph nodes, pericolic: Negative for metastasis (0/6)

Pericolic adipose: Metastatic adenocarcinoma

II. Liver (needle biopsy): Metastatic adenocarcinoma

Case 2: Solution

1.   Principal diagnosis: _____

_____

2.   Other diagnoses: _____

_____

3.   Procedures: _____

_____

4.   Issues to clarify with physician: _____

_____

Case 3

Emergency Department Record

Chief Complaint: Shortness of breath

History of Present Illness: This is a 72-year-old male with a long history of bullous emphysema. He has home breathing treatments and is on Aminophylline and Lanoxin and pO_2 11/2 liters pm at home. Patient presents with a two-day history of increasing dyspnea, and became increasingly restless and short of breath tonight. He was brought in here by family for evaluation. He does complain of feeling hot but denies any chills or increasing cough recently. Patient also has a history of CHF per his wife.

Physical Examination: Vital signs, temperature not recorded, pulse 135, respirations 32, blood pressure 124/82. Patient is cyanotic at the fingertips and somewhat dusky. He is breathing with pursed lips at a rapid rate and sitting up. Lung exam demonstrated very poor air movement bilaterally. Cardiac exam was irregular rhythm without murmurs, rubs, or gallops, and was tachycardiac. The patient has extremely dry leatherlike skin with brownish discoloration in the pretibial area, along with some scaling and chronic skin changes.

Initial ABG, which was obtained immediately on 2 liters of oxygen, showed a pH of 7.15, pCO_2 of 69.5, pO_2 of 50, and bicarb of 25.5 with 72% oxygen saturation. Initially we gave him 2 breathing treatments over 45 minutes consisting of Albuterol med/neb along with Solu-Medrol 125 mg IV push and 2 liters of oxygen support, hoping that he would improve and we could avoid intubation. However, during this 45-minute period the patient started developing multi-focal PVCs and also had runs of 3, 4, and 5 PVCs at a time, but had no chest pain. Therefore, we increased the patient's oxygen and placed him on lidocaine of 75 mg IV push bolus along with lidocaine at 2 mg per minute, resulting in good resolution of his arrhythmia except for a rare PVC. We did repeat his ABG while on 40% mask, which showed a pH of 7.17, pCO_2 of 75, pO_2 of 72, and bicarb of 2.8 at 89%.

Due to the extreme acidosis and the tachypnea, I discussed with the family (the patient and his wife, 2 sons, and also a son over the phone) that we should intubate the patient before he had impending respiratory failure.

The patient was therefore intubated per respiratory with number 8 ET tube. Ventilation was initially set on tidal volume of 500 cc with a rate of 16. Repeat gases on this after a half hour showed a pH of 7.15, pCO_2 of 68, pO_2 of 66, bicarb of 25, and O_2 sat of 85%. We therefore increased his tidal volume of 600 cc and kept him on the vent. A portable chest x-ray was done after tube placement, which showed the tube to be in excellent placement. Laboratory data included a hemoglobin of 18.6, hematocrit 58.1, white count 7,400 with 4 bands, 54 segs, CPK was high at 259, and MB was pending. EKG showed multi-focal PVCs and atrial fibrillation with a rapid ventricular rate. Theophylline level was 11.6, Lanoxin level was 1.

History

Chief Complaint: Shortness of breath, restlessness, tingling in the hands, swelling of the feet

History of Present Illness: This 72-year-old white male has a history of rather advanced chronic obstructive pulmonary disease for many years. He presented to the Emergency Department with progressive dyspnea of two days' duration, restlessness, and feeling hot and burning up. According to his wife, the patient had episodes where he suddenly became dyspneic, was turning red all over, and had tingling all over his body. He did not have a cold or fever. He was evaluated in the Emergency Department. Patient had evidence of respiratory acidosis with respiratory failure with a pH of 7.15, pCO_2 of 68, pO_2 of 66, bicarb of 12, O_2 saturation of 85%. The patient was markedly dyspneic with labored respirations. Hemoglobin was 18.6 grams. EKG showed premature ectopic beats. Theophylline level was 7.6, Dig level was 1.0.

The patient was intubated and transferred to ICU for further care. It was felt at that time that respiratory acidosis may have contributed to the patient's ectopy and the deterioration of his clinical condition. The patient was initially given respiratory therapy in the Emergency Department without any significant improvement.

The patient has a history of rather advanced chronic obstructive pulmonary disease with bullous emphysema. He also has a history of congestive cardiac failure with cor pulmonale. The patient has been on home IPPB treatment. He has also been on bronchodilators, intermittent antibiotic therapy, and O_2 therapy at home. He also has venous insufficiency in the lower extremities and stasis ulcer in the left leg, which has been healing slowly with local treatment and systemic antibiotic therapy.

Past Medical History: The patient was hospitalized for prostate surgery many years ago. He also has had a cataract removed with intraocular implant. A year ago, he had a skin lesion removed from the nose, which was basal cell carcinoma. He was treated with local radiation therapy.

Family History: Noncontributory

Personal History: He is married. He quit smoking cigarettes approximately 12 years ago. Drinks alcohol occasionally. Drinks 4–5 cups of coffee a day.

Review of Systems: Unremarkable, except for present illness

Physical Examination

The patient is a well-developed, well-nourished white male in acute respiratory distress, markedly cyanotic with labored respirations. He is slightly lethargic. BP is 130/86, Pulse 110; respirations were 38.

Head: Unremarkable.

Eyes: Evidence of surgery from previous cataract surgery with intraocular implant. No other abnormalities.

ENT: The patient is intubated with ET tube inserted. Copious secretions from the oral cavity. Surgical scar on nose from previous surgery.

Neck: Shows no masses, no venous engorgement, no bruit.

Chest: Air entry is equal on both sides. Scattered rhonchi both lung fields with minimal diffuse basilar rales.

Heart: Irregular rhythm with ectopy. A Grade H x VI apical murmur present.

Abdomen: Soft, no tenderness. No palpable masses. Bowel sounds active. Hernia. Orifices normal.

Rectal Exam: Deferred.

Extremities: Edema in both lower extremities with marked excoriation and scaling of the skin distal to the knee with an ulcerative lesion in the left leg with hyperpigmentation for the skin of both lower extremities without any signs of acute infection.

Impression: Clinically, the patient has stasis dermatitis; stasis ulcer also in the left leg.

Neurological exam is consistent with mild peripheral neuropathy.

Consultation

Patient has several-day history of increasing amounts of shortness of breath, increasing sputum production, and increased complaints of feeling hot, but denied chills. Patient was admitted for acute shortness of breath, respiratory failure needing intubation and respiratory and ventilator care now.

Apparently, the patient came to the hospital with no chest pain, but having occasional and/or frequent PVCs requiring lidocaine initiation as well as increased amounts of oxygen. Secondary to respiratory acidosis, the patient was intubated. ABGs are to follow. Patient has a long history of emphysema with bullous changes in his lungs. He has a history of congestive heart failure as well as potential cardiac dysrhythmia. The patient currently is on ventilator care and was extubated yesterday. Postextubation, apparently 8 hrs later patient had fatigue requiring reintubation noted. Other past medical history is significant of having extremity varicosities as well as ulceration and senile dementia. Patient has no known allergies.

Laboratory investigations of ABGs show acute respiratory acidosis, hypoxemia increased AA gradient noted. Subsequent arterial blood gases have been done with the patient on the ventilator. Patient's EKG showed that of sinus tachycardia with sinus arrhythmia. Some PVCs noted on the occasional EKG.

Patient has been in atrial fibrillation intermittently. His x-rays show bilateral hyperinflated airways. The patient does have a large left heart with some nonspecific interstitial markings. Patient appears to have fibrotic changes. No pleural effusion in the patient's left base. Review of chest x-ray changes shows some increase in the interstitial markings. Left heart remains enlarged.

Consulting Diagnoses:

1. Acute exacerbation of COPD emphysema in stages leading to respiratory failure that of acute respiratory acidosis and hypoxemia
2. Probable superimposed upon respiratory failure with COPD emphysema is that of cardiac dysrhythmia and probable mild to moderate congestive heart failure
3. Probable significant coronary artery disease and cor pulmonale, II
4. Theophylline toxic at this time

Laboratory Tests

Test	1/9	1/9	1/9	1/9	Reference
ART BLOOD GASES					
pH	7.154 L		7.167 L	7.152 L	7.340–7.450
pCO_2	69.5 H		74.9 H	67.9 H	32.0–5.0
pO_2	50.2 L		72.0 L	66.1 L	75.0–100.0
Bicarb	23.4		26.1 H	22.8	20.0–26.0
Total CO_2	25.5		28.4 H	24.9	21.0–27.0
O_2 sat	72.5 L		88.5 L	85.2 L	95.0–98.0
CHEMISTRY					
Glucose		157 H			77–115
BUN		23			8–24
Creatinine		1.4 H			0.5–1.2
Sodium		141			137–147
Potassium		4.6			3.6–5.2
Chloride		103			97–111
CO_2		31			21–32
CK Total		259 H			55–215
CKMB		3.3			0.4–4.7
LDH		173			91–179
SGOT-AST		45 H			11–33
Magnesium		1.8			1.6–2.4
THERAPEUTIC DRUGS					
Digoxin		1.0			0.8–1.6
Theophylline		11.6			10.0–20.0

Laboratory Tests

Test	1/12	1/12	1/13	1/13	Reference
ART BLOOD GASES					
pH	7.419	7.434		7.477 H	7.340–7.450
pCO_2	42.6	41.3		41.0	32.0–45.0
pO_2	52.7 L	51.3 L		57.0 L	75.0–100.0
Bicarb	27.4 H	27.5 H		30.2 H	20.0–26.0
Total CO_2	28.7 H	28.7 H		31.5	21.0–27.0
O_2 sat	87.5 L	87.2 L		91.3 L	95.0–98.0
CHEMISTRY					
Potassium			3.2 L		3.6–5.2
THERAPEUTIC DRUGS					
Theophylline			34.1 H		10.0–20.0

Clinical Resume

This 72-year-old white male has history of fairly advanced chronic obstructive pulmonary disease for many years. He presented to the emergency department with progressive shortness of breath of several days' duration, associated with restlessness, feeling hot, and burning up. He did not have any history of recent cold, fever, or flu. He had several episodes of acute shortness of breath prior to admission. He was evaluated in the Emergency Department and was in acute respiratory failure with pH of 7.15, pCO_2 of 68, and pO_2 of 66. Saturation was 85%. The patient was intubated in the Emergency Department and transferred to ICU for further care. His hemoglobin was 18.6 grams. EKG showed premature ventricular ectopic beats. Theophylline level was 11.6. Digoxin level was 1.0. The patient has history of chronic obstructive pulmonary disease with bullous emphysema. He also has history of congestive heart failure. He has been on bronchodilators, IPPB, intermittent antibiotic therapy at home. In addition to the above, he has venous insufficiency in both lower extremities with stasis dermatitis and stasis ulcers in the lower extremity.

On physical examination, he was a well-developed, well-nourished white male in acute respiratory distress with labored respiration, slightly lethargic. BP 130/86, pulse 110, resp 38. Examination of the HEENT, neck was unremarkable. Chest showed bilateral rhonchi in both lung fields with minimal diffuse basilar rales. Heart rhythm was irregular with ectopy. Grade II by VI apical murmur was present. Abdominal examination was unremarkable. Extremities showed edema in both lower extremities and marked excoriation and scaling of the skin distal to the knee, ulcerative lesions in the left leg with hyperpigmentation consistent with stasis dermatitis.

Laboratory Data: Chest x-ray showed no acute infiltrate. There was a suggestion of mild congestive cardiac failure. EKG showed atrial fibrillation with ventricular ectopic beats and showed lateral ischemia. Arterial blood gases showed pH of 7.15, pCO_2 of 69.5, and pO_2 of 50. Blood glucose was 157, BUN 23, and creatinine 1.4. Electrolytes were normal. Digoxin level was 1.0. Theophylline was 11.6.

Course in Hospital: The patient was intubated and transferred to ICU, where he was started on ventilatory support. He was seen later on the same day with marked improvement in his clinical condition. He was more alert and responsive, and there was also improvement in the acidosis. He was continued on the same therapy. On 1-11, the patient was reevaluated. He had significant improvement. His acidosis had been corrected, and ABGs showed a pO_2 of 55 and pCO_2 of 59 with good negative inspiratory effort. It was felt that the patient could tolerate extubation. He was extubated on 1-11. He tolerated it well for 6 hrs. post extubation. Subsequent to that, he developed gradual increasing pCO_2 and decreasing pO_2 with acidosis. His respirations became labored and the patient became cyanotic. He was reintubated on January 11 and started on ventilatory support.

The next day, the patient was clinically improved. His vital signs were also improved. A consultation was obtained from a pulmonologist. In his opinion, the patient had respiratory failure with acute exacerbation of chronic obstructive pulmonary disease. When he examined the patient, the patient's Theophylline was higher than therapeutic level, at 34.1. He recommended that the patient be continued on ventilatory support. Electrolyte imbalance should be corrected and also his dose of Theophylline needed adjustment. All these orders were carried out. The patient started showing signs of improvement. When the patient's condition was stable, he was started on intermittent ventilation. He had signs of congestive cardiac failure, which were treated with diuretics. He was continued on Digoxin. Patient was extubated on January 15. This time he tolerated it well. His condition remained stable and he was transferred to a regular unit. He was initially placed on corticosteroids. The dose was gradually decreased, and he was switched to oral antibiotics and corticosteroids. He continued to improve but still was dyspneic. However, he was markedly improved since admission.

After he recovered to a significant level and his oral intake had improved, pulmonary rehabilitation was discussed with the patient. It is felt that the patient could be discharged at this time and be followed up as an outpatient. After the patient was informed that he would be discharged that morning, he became anxious, agitated, and very apprehensive. Arterial blood gases were still satisfactory for a patient who has chronic obstructive pulmonary disease. His pCO_2 level was 71.2, pO_2 was 77.3, and pH was 7.3. It was discovered that there was an element of anxiety on the patient's part, and he may require further supportive care. However, continuation of hospitalization would not benefit the patient. He was discharged on 1/23. At the time of discharge, the patient had mild dyspnea. However, he had significantly improved. His vital signs were stable.

Medications at Discharge:

1. No-added-salt diet with high-fat and low-carbohydrate content
2. Procardia SR 500 mg tid
3. Slobid 200 mg bid
4. Lasix 40 mg daily
5. Zantac 150 mg daily
6. Lanoxin .25 mg daily except on Sunday
7. K-Dur 20 mg daily
8. Prednisone 20 mg twice a day for four days; once a day for one week; and 10 mg daily for one week and 10 mg every day subsequent to that

Case 3: Solution

1. Principal diagnosis: _____

   _____

2. Other diagnoses: _____

   _____

3. Procedures: _____

   _____

4. Issues to clarify with physician: _____

   _____

Appendix A

AHIMA Code of Ethics

Preamble

The ethical obligations of the health information management (HIM) professional include the protection of patient privacy and confidential information; disclosure of information; development, use, and maintenance of health information systems and health records; and the quality of information. Both handwritten and computerized medical records contain many sacred stories—stories that must be protected on behalf of the individual and the aggregate community of persons served in the healthcare system. Healthcare consumers are increasingly concerned about the loss of privacy and the inability to control the dissemination of their protected information. Core health information issues include what information should be collected; how the information should be handled, who should have access to the information, and under what conditions the information should be disclosed.

Ethical obligations are central to the professional's responsibility, regardless of the employment site or the method of collection, storage, and security of health information. Sensitive information (genetic, adoption, drug, alcohol, sexual, and behavioral information) requires special attention to prevent misuse. Entrepreneurial roles require expertise in the protection of the information in the world of business and interactions with consumers.

Professional Values

The mission of the HIM profession is based on core professional values developed since the inception of the Association in 1928. These values and the inherent ethical responsibilities for AHIMA members and credentialed HIM professionals include providing service, protecting medical, social, and financial information, promoting confidentiality; and preserving and securing health information. Values to the healthcare team include promoting the quality and advancement of healthcare, demonstrating HIM expertise and skills, and promoting interdisciplinary cooperation and collaboration. Professional values in relationship to the employer include protecting committee deliberations and complying with laws, regulations, and policies. Professional values related to the public include advocating change, refusing to participate or conceal unethical practices, and reporting violations of practice standards to the proper authorities. Professional

Source: Revised & adopted by AHIMA House of Delegates, July 1, 2004.

149

values to individual and professional associations include obligations to be honest, bringing honor to self, peers and profession, committing to continuing education and lifelong learning, performing Association duties honorably, strengthening professional membership, representing the profession to the public, and promoting and participating in research.

These professional values will require a complex process of balancing the many conflicts that can result from competing interests and obligations of those who seek access to health information and require an understanding of ethical decision-making.

Purpose of the American Health Information Management Association Code of Ethics

The HIM professional has an obligation to demonstrate actions that reflect values, ethical principles, and ethical guidelines. The American Health Information Management Association (AHIMA) Code of Ethics sets forth these values and principles to guide conduct. The code is relevant to all AHIMA members and credentialed HIM professionals and students, regardless of their professional functions, the settings in which they work, or the populations they serve.

The AHIMA Code of Ethics serves six purposes:

- Identifies core values on which the HIM mission is based.

- Summarizes broad ethical principles that reflect the profession's core values and establishes a set of ethical principles to be used to guide decision-making and actions.

- Helps HIM professionals identify relevant considerations when professional obligations conflict or ethical uncertainties arise.

- Provides ethical principles by which the general public can hold the HIM professional accountable.

- Socializes practitioners new to the field to HIM's mission, values, and ethical principles.

- Articulates a set of guidelines that the HIM professional can use to assess whether they have engaged in unethical conduct.

The code includes principles and guidelines that are both enforceable and aspirational. The extent to which each principle is enforceable is a matter of professional judgment to be exercised by those responsible for reviewing alleged violations of ethical principles.

The Use of the Code

Violation of principles in this code does not automatically imply legal liability or violation of the law. Such determination can only be made in the context of legal and judicial proceedings. Alleged violations of the code would be subject to a peer review process. Such processes are generally separate from legal or administrative procedures and insulated from legal review or proceedings to allow the profession to counsel and discipline its own members although in some situations, violations of the code would constitute unlawful conduct subject to legal process.

Guidelines for ethical and unethical behavior are provided in this code. The terms "shall and shall not" are used as a basis for setting high standards for behavior. This does not imply that everyone "shall or shall not" do everything that is listed. For example, not everyone participates in the recruitment or mentoring of students. A HIM professional is not being unethical if this is not part of his or her professional activities; however, if students are part of one's professional responsibilities, there is an ethical obligation to follow the guidelines stated in the code. This concept is true for the entire code. If someone does the stated activities, ethical behavior is the standard. The guidelines are not a comprehensive list. For example, the statement "protect all confidential information to include personal, health, financial, genetic and outcome information" can also be interpreted as "shall not fail to protect all confidential information to include personal, health, financial, genetic, and outcome information."

A code of ethics cannot guarantee ethical behavior. Moreover, a code of ethics cannot resolve all ethical issues or disputes or capture the richness and complexity involved in striving to make responsible choices within a moral community. Rather, a code of ethics sets forth values and ethical principles, and offers ethical guidelines to which professionals aspire and by which their actions can be judged. Ethical behaviors result from a personal commitment to engage in ethical practice.

Professional responsibilities often require an individual to move beyond personal values. For example, an individual might demonstrate behaviors that are based on the values of honesty, providing service to others, or demonstrating loyalty. In addition to these, professional values might require promoting confidentiality, facilitating interdisciplinary collaboration, and refusing to participate or conceal unethical practices. Professional values could require a more comprehensive set of values than what an individual needs to be an ethical agent in their personal lives.

The AHIMA Code of Ethics is to be used by AHIMA and individuals, agencies, organizations, and bodies (such as licensing and regulatory boards, insurance providers, courts of law, agency boards of directors, government agencies, and other professional groups) that choose to adopt it or use it as a frame of reference. The AHIMA Code of Ethics reflects the commitment of all to uphold the profession's values and to act ethically. Individuals of good character who discern moral questions and, in good faith, seek to make reliable ethical judgments, must apply ethical principles.

The code does not provide a set of rules that prescribe how to act in all situations. Specific applications of the code must take into account the context in which it is being considered and the possibility of conflicts among the code's values, principles, and guidelines. Ethical responsibilities flow from all human relationships, from the personal and familial to the social and professional. Further, the AHIMA Code of Ethics does not specify which values, principles, and guidelines are the most important and ought to outweigh others in instances when they conflict.

Code of Ethics 2004

Ethical Principles: The following ethical principles are based on the core values of the American Health Information Management Association and apply to all health information management professionals.

Health information management professionals:

    I. *Advocate, uphold and defend the individual's right to privacy and the doctrine of confidentiality in the use and disclosure of information.*

    II. *Put service and the health and welfare of persons before self-interest and conduct themselves in the practice of the profession so as to bring honor to themselves, their peers, and to the health information management profession.*

    III. *Preserve, protect, and secure personal health information in any form or medium and hold in the highest regard the contents of the records and other information of a confidential nature, taking into account the applicable statutes and regulations.*

    IV. *Refuse to participate in or conceal unethical practices or procedures.*

    V. *Advance health information management knowledge and practice through continuing education, research, publications, and presentations.*

    VI. *Recruit and mentor students, peers and colleagues to develop and strengthen professional workforce.*

    VII. *Accurately represent the profession to the public.*

    VIII. *Perform honorably health information management association responsibilities, either appointed or elected, and preserve the confidentiality of any privileged information made known in any official capacity.*

    IX. *State truthfully and accurately their credentials, professional education, and experiences.*

    X. *Facilitate interdisciplinary collaboration in situations supporting health information practice.*

    XI. *Respect the inherent dignity and worth of every person.*

How to Interpret the Code of Ethics

The following ethical principles are based on the core values of the American Health Information Management Association and apply to all health information management professionals. Guidelines included for each ethical principle are a non-inclusive list of behaviors and situations that can help to clarify the principle. They are not to be meant as a comprehensive list of all situations that can occur.

    I. *Advocate, uphold, and defend the individual's right to privacy and the doctrine of confidentiality in the use and disclosure of information.*

Health information management professionals **shall**:

1.1. Protect all confidential information to include personal, health, financial, genetic, and outcome information.

1.2. Engage in social and political action that supports the protection of privacy and confidentiality, and be aware of the impact of the political arena on the health information system. Advocate for changes in policy and legislation to ensure protection of privacy and confidentiality, coding compliance, and other issues that surface as advocacy issues as well as facilitating informed participation by the public on these issues.

1.3. Protect the confidentiality of all information obtained in the course of professional service. Disclose only information that is directly relevant or necessary to achieve the purpose of disclosure. Release information only with valid consent from a patient or a person legally authorized to consent on behalf of a patient or as authorized by federal or state regulations. The need-to-know criterion is essential when releasing health information for initial disclosure and all redisclosure activities.

1.4. Promote the obligation to respect privacy by respecting confidential information shared among colleagues, while responding to requests from the legal profession, the media, or other non-healthcare related individuals, during presentations or teaching and in situations that could cause harm to persons.

II. Put service and the health and welfare of persons before self-interest and conduct themselves in the practice of the profession so as to bring honor to themselves, their peers, and to the health information management profession.

Health information management professionals **shall**:

2.1. Act with integrity, behave in a trustworthy manner, elevate service to others above self-interest, and promote high standards of practice in every setting.

2.2. Be aware of the profession's mission, values, and ethical principles, and practice in a manner consistent with them by acting honestly and responsibly.

2.3. Anticipate, clarify, and avoid any conflict of interest, to all parties concerned, when dealing with consumers, consulting with competitors, or in providing services requiring potentially conflicting roles (for example, finding out information about one facility that would help a competitor). The conflicting roles or responsibilities must be clarified and appropriate action must be taken to minimize any conflict of interest.

2.4. Ensure that the working environment is consistent and encourages compliance with the AHIMA Code of Ethics, taking reasonable steps to eliminate any conditions in their organizations that violate, interfere with, or discourage compliance with the code.

2.5. Take responsibility and credit, including authorship credit, only for work they actually perform or to which they contribute. Honestly acknowledge the work of and the contributions made by others verbally or written, such as in publication.

Health information management professionals **shall not**:

2.6. Permit their private conduct to interfere with their ability to fulfill their professional responsibilities.

2.7. Take unfair advantage of any professional relationship or exploit others to further their personal, religious, political, or business interests.

III. Preserve, protect, and secure personal health information in any form or medium and hold in the highest regard the contents of the records and other information of a confidential nature, taking into account the applicable statutes and regulations.

Health information management professionals **shall**:

3.1. Protect the confidentiality of patients' written and electronic records and other sensitive information. Take reasonable steps to ensure that patients' records are stored in a secure location and that patients' records are not available to others who are not authorized to have access.

3.2. Take precautions to ensure and maintain the confidentiality of information transmitted, transferred, or disposed of in the event of a termination, incapacitation, or death of a healthcare provider to other parties through the use of any media. Disclosure of identifying information should be avoided whenever possible.

3.3. Inform recipients of the limitations and risks associated with providing services via electronic media (such as computer, telephone, fax, radio, and television).

IV. *Refuse to participate in or conceal unethical practices or procedures.*

Health information management professionals **shall:**

4.1. Act in a professional and ethical manner at all times.

4.2. Take adequate measures to discourage, prevent, expose, and correct the unethical conduct of colleagues.

4.3. Be knowledgeable about established policies and procedures for handling concerns about colleagues' unethical behavior. These include policies and procedures created by AHIMA, licensing and regulatory bodies, employers, supervisors, agencies, and other professional organizations.

4.4. Seek resolution if there is a belief that a colleague has acted unethically or if there is a belief of incompetence or impairment by discussing their concerns with the colleague when feasible and when such discussion is likely to be productive. Take action through appropriate formal channels, such as contacting an accreditation or regulatory body and/ or the AHIMA Professional Ethics Committee.

4.5. Consult with a colleague when feasible and assist the colleague in taking remedial action when there is direct knowledge of a health information management colleague's incompetence or impairment.

Health information management professionals **shall not**:

4.6. Participate in, condone, or be associated with dishonesty, fraud and abuse, or deception. A non-inclusive list of examples includes:

- Allowing patterns of retrospective documentation to avoid suspension or increase reimbursement

- Assigning codes without physician documentation

- Coding when documentation does not justify the procedures that have been billed

- Coding an inappropriate level of service

- Miscoding to avoid conflict with others

- Engaging in negligent coding practices

- Hiding or ignoring review outcomes, such as performance data

- Failing to report licensure status for a physician through the appropriate channels

- Recording inaccurate data for accreditation purposes

- Hiding incomplete medical records

- Allowing inappropriate access to genetic, adoption, or behavioral health information

- Misusing sensitive information about a competitor

- Violating the privacy of individuals

V. **Advance health information management knowledge and practice through continuing education, research, publications, and presentations.**

Health information management professionals **shall**:

5.1. Develop and enhance continually their professional expertise, knowledge, and skills (including appropriate education, research, training, consultation, and supervision). Contribute to the knowledge base of health information management and share with colleagues their knowledge related to practice, research, and ethics.

5.2. Base practice decisions on recognized knowledge, including empirically based knowledge relevant to health information management and health information management ethics.

5.3. Contribute time and professional expertise to activities that promote respect for the value, integrity, and competence of the health information management profession. These activities may include teaching, research, consultation, service, legislative testimony, presentations in the community, and participation in their professional organizations.

5.4. Engage in evaluation or research that ensures the anonymity or confidentiality of participants and of the data obtained from them by following guidelines developed for the participants in consultation with appropriate institutional review boards. Report evaluation and research findings accurately and take steps to correct any errors later found in published data using standard publication methods.

5.5. Take reasonable steps to provide or arrange for continuing education and staff development, addressing current knowledge and emerging developments related to health information management practice and ethics.

Health information management professionals **shall not**:

5.6. Design or conduct evaluation or research that is in conflict with applicable federal or state laws.

5.7. Participate in, condone, or be associated with fraud or abuse.

VI. **Recruit and mentor students, peers and colleagues to develop and strengthen professional workforce.**

Health information management professionals **shall**:

6.1. Evaluate students' performance in a manner that is fair and respectful when functioning as educators or clinical internship supervisors.

6.2. Be responsible for setting clear, appropriate, and culturally sensitive boundaries for students.

6.3. Be a mentor for students, peers and new health information management professionals to develop and strengthen skills.

6.4. Provide directed practice opportunities for students.

Health information management professionals **shall not**:

6.5. Engage in any relationship with students in which there is a risk of exploitation or potential harm to the student.

VII. *Accurately represent the profession to the public.*

Health information management professionals **shall:**

7.1 Be an advocate for the profession in all settings and participate in activities that promote and explain the mission, values, and principles of the profession to the public.

VIII. *Perform honorably health information management association responsibilities, either appointed or elected, and preserve the confidentiality of any privileged information made known in any official capacity.*

Health information management professionals **shall:**

8.1. Perform responsibly all duties as assigned by the professional association.

8.2. Resign from an Association position if unable to perform the assigned responsibilities with competence.

8.3. Speak on behalf of professional health information management organizations, accurately representing the official and authorized positions of the organizations.

IX. *State truthfully and accurately their credentials, professional education, and experiences.*

Health information management professionals **shall:**

9.1. Make clear distinctions between statements made and actions engaged in as a private individual and as a representative of the health information management profession, a professional health information organization, or the health information management professional's employer.

9.2. Claim and ensure that their representations to patients, agencies, and the public of professional qualifications, credentials, education, competence, affiliations, services provided, training, certification, consultation received, supervised experience, other relevant professional experience are accurate.

9.3. Claim only those relevant professional credentials actually possessed and correct any inaccuracies occurring regarding credentials.

X. *Facilitate interdisciplinary collaboration in situations supporting health information practice.*

Health information management professionals **shall:**

10.1. Participate in and contribute to decisions that affect the well-being of patients by drawing on the perspectives, values, and experiences of those involved in decisions related to patients. Professional and ethical obligations of the interdisciplinary team as a whole and of its individual members should be clearly established.

XI. *Respect the inherent dignity and worth of every person.*

Health information management professionals **shall:**

11.1. Treat each person in a respectful fashion, being mindful of individual differences and cultural and ethnic diversity.

11.2. Promote the value of self-determination for each individual.

Acknowledgement

Adapted with permission from the Code of Ethics of the National Association of Social Workers.

Resources

National Association of Social Workers. 1999. Code of ethics. Available online from http://www.naswdc.org/pubs/code/code.asp.

Harman, L.B. (Ed.). 2001. *Ethical Challenges in the Management of Health Information.* Aspen: Gaithersburg, MD.

AHIMA Code of Ethics, 1957, 1977, 1988, and 1998.

Appendix B

AHIMA Practice Brief: Developing a Coding Compliance Policy Document

Organizations using diagnosis and procedure codes for reporting healthcare services must have formal policies and corresponding procedures in place that provide instruction on the entire process—from the point of service to the billing statement or claim form. Coding compliance policies serve as a guide to performing coding and billing functions and provide documentation of the organization's intent to correctly report services. The policies should include facility-specific documentation requirements, payer regulations and policies, and contractual arrangements for coding consultants and outsourcing services. This information may be covered in payer/provider contracts or found in Medicare and Medicaid manuals and bulletins.

Following are selected tenets that address the process of code selection and reporting. These tenets may be referred to as coding protocols, a coding compliance program, organizational coding guidelines, or a similar name. These tenets are an important part of any organization's compliance plan and the key to preventing coding errors and resulting reimbursement problems. Examples are taken from both outpatient and inpatient coding processes for illustration purposes only. This document cannot serve as a complete coding compliance plan, but will be useful as a guide for creating a more comprehensive resource to meet individual organizational needs.

A coding compliance plan should include the following components:

- A general policy statement about the commitment of the organization to correctly assign and report codes

    Example: Memorial Medical Center is committed to establishing and maintaining clinical coding and insurance claims processing procedures to ensure that reported codes reflect actual services provided, through accurate information system entries.

- The source of the official coding guidelines used to direct code selection

    Example: ICD-9-CM code selection follows the Official Guidelines for Coding and Reporting, developed by the cooperating parties and documented in *Coding Clinic for ICD-9-CM,* published by the American Hospital Association.

    Example: CPT code selection follows the guidelines set forth in the CPT manual and in *CPT Assistant,* published by the American Medical Association.

Source: AHIMA Coding Practice Team. 2001 (July/August). Practice brief: Developing a coding compliance policy document. *Journal of American Health Information Management Association* 72(7):88A–C.

- The parties responsible for code assignment. The ultimate responsibility for code assignment lies with the physician (provider). However, policies and procedures may document instances where codes may be selected or modified by authorized individuals

  Example: For inpatient records, medical record analyst I staff are responsible for analysis of records and assignment of the correct ICD-9-CM codes based on documentation by the attending physician.

  Example: Emergency department evaluation and management levels for physician services will be selected by the physician and validated by outpatient record analysts using the HCFA/AMA documentation guidelines. When a variance occurs, the following steps are taken for resolution (The actual document should follow with procedure details).

- The procedure to follow when the clinical information is not clear enough to assign the correct code

  Example: When the documentation used to assign codes is ambiguous or incomplete, the physician must be contacted to clarify the information and complete/amend the record, if necessary. (The actual document should follow with details of how the medical staff would like this to occur, e.g., by phone call, by note on the record, etc.). Standard protocols for adding documentation to a record must be followed, in accordance with the applicable laws and regulations.

- Specify the policies and procedures that apply to specific locations and care settings. Official coding guidelines for inpatient reporting and outpatient/physician reporting are different. This means that if you are developing a facility-specific coding guideline for emergency department services, designate that the coding rules or guidelines only apply in this setting

  Example: When reporting an injection of a drug provided in the emergency department to a Medicare beneficiary, the appropriate CPT code for the administration of the injection is reported in addition to the evaluation and management service code and drug code. CPT codes are reported whether a physician provides the injection personally or a nurse is carrying out a physician's order. This instruction does not always apply for reporting of professional services in the clinics, because administration of medication is considered bundled with the corresponding evaluation and management service for Medicare patients.

  Example: Diagnoses that are documented as "probable," "suspected," "questionable," "rule-out," or "working diagnosis" are not to have a code assigned as a confirmed diagnosis. Instead, the code for the condition established at the close of the encounter should be assigned, such as a symptom, sign, abnormal test result, or clinical finding. This guideline applies only to outpatient services.

- Applicable reporting requirements required by specific agencies. The document should include where instructions on payer-specific requirements may be accessed

  Example: For patients with XYZ care plan, report code S0800 for patients having a LASIK procedure rather than an unlisted CPT code.

  Example: For Medicare patients receiving a wound closure by tissue adhesive only, report HCPCS Level II code G0168 rather than a CPT code.

Many of these procedures will be put into software databases and would not be written as a specific policy. This is true with most billing software, whether for physician services or through the charge description master used by many hospitals.

- Procedures for correction of inaccurate code assignments in the clinical database and to the agencies where the codes have been reported

    Example: When an error in code assignment is discovered after bill release and the claim has already been submitted, this is the process required to update and correct the information system and facilitate claim amendment or correction (The actual document should follow with appropriate details).

- Areas of risk that have been identified through audits or monitoring. Each organization should have a defined audit plan for code accuracy and consistency review and corrective actions should be outlined for problems that are identified

    Example: A hospital might identify that acute respiratory failure is being assigned as the principal diagnosis with congestive heart failure as a secondary diagnosis. The specific reference to *Coding Clinic* could be listed with instructions about correct coding of these conditions and the process to be used to correct the deficiency.

- Identification of essential coding resources available to and used by the coding professionals

    Example: Updated ICD-9-CM, CPT, and HCPCS Level II code books are used by all coding professionals. Even if the hospital uses automated encoding software, at least one printed copy of the coding manuals should be available for reference.

    Example: Updated encoder software, including the appropriate version of the NCCI edits and DRG and APC grouper software, is available to the appropriate personnel.

    Example: *Coding Clinic* and *CPT Assistant* are available to all coding professionals.

- A process for coding new procedures or unusual diagnoses

    Example: When the coding professional encounters an unusual diagnosis, the coding supervisor or the attending physician is consulted. If, after research, a code cannot be identified, the documentation is submitted to the AHA for clarification.

- A procedure to identify any optional codes gathered for statistical purposes by the facility and clarification of the appropriate use of E codes

    Example: All ICD-9-CM procedure codes in the surgical range (ICD-9-CM Volume III codes 01.01-86.99) shall be reported for inpatients. In addition, codes reported from the non-surgical section include the following (Completed document should list the actual codes to be reported).

    Example: All appropriate E codes for adverse effects of drugs must be reported. In addition, this facility reports all E codes, including the place of injury for poisonings, all cases of abuse, and all accidents on the initial visit for both inpatient and outpatient services.

- Appropriate methods for resolving coding or documentation disputes with physicians

  Example: When the physician disagrees with official coding guidelines, the case is referred to the medical records committee following review by the designated physician liaison from that group.

- A procedure for processing claim rejections

  Example: All rejected claims pertaining to diagnosis and procedure codes should be returned to coding staff for review or correction. Any chargemaster issues should be forwarded to appropriate departmental staff for corrections. All clinical codes, including modifiers, must never be changed or added without review by coding staff with access to the appropriate documentation.

  Example: If a claim is rejected due to the codes provided in the medical record abstract, the billing department notifies the supervisor of coding for a review rather than changing the code to a payable code and resubmitting the claim.

- A statement clarifying that codes will not be assigned, modified, or excluded solely for the purpose of maximizing reimbursement. Clinical codes will not be changed or amended merely due to either physicians' or patients' request to have the service in question covered by insurance. If the initial code assignment did not reflect the actual services, codes may be revised based on supporting documentation. Disputes with either physicians or patients are handled only by the coding supervisor and are appropriately logged for review

  Example: A patient calls the business office saying that her insurance carrier did not pay for her mammogram. After investigating, the HIM coding staff discover that the coding was appropriate for a screening mammogram and that this is a non-covered service with the insurance provider. The code is not changed and the matter is referred back to the business office for explanation to the patient that she should contact her insurance provider with any dispute over coverage of service.

  Example: Part of a payment is denied and after review, the supervisor discovers that a modifier should have been appended to the CPT code to denote a separately identifiable service. Modifier –25 is added to the code set and the corrected claim is resubmitted.

  Example: A physician approaches the coding supervisor with a request to change the diagnosis codes for his patient because what she currently has is a pre-existing condition that is not covered by her current health plan. The coding supervisor must explain to the physician that falsification of insurance claims is illegal. If the physician insists, the physician liaison for the medical record committee is contacted and the matter is turned over to that committee for resolution if necessary.

- The use of and reliance on encoders within the organization. Coding staff cannot rely solely on computerized encoders. Current coding manuals must be readily accessible and the staff must be educated appropriately to detect inappropriate logic or errors in encoding software. When errors in logic or code crosswalks are discovered, they are reported to the vendor immediately by the coding supervisor

  Example: During the coding process, an error is identified in the crosswalk between the ICD-9-CM Volume III code and the CPT code. This error is reported to the software vendor, with proper documentation and notification of all staff using the encoder to not rely on the encoder for code selection.

- Medical records are analyzed and codes selected only with complete and appropriate documentation by the physician available. According to coding guidelines, codes are not assigned without physician documentation. If records are coded without the discharge summary or final diagnostic statements available, processes are in place for review after the summary is added to the record

  Example: When records are coded without a discharge summary, they are flagged in the computer system. When the summaries are added to the record, the record is returned to the coding professional for review of codes. If there are any inconsistencies, appropriate steps are taken for review of the changes.

Additional Elements

A coding compliance document should include a reference to the AHIMA Standards of Ethical Coding, which can be downloaded from AHIMA's Web site at www.ahima.org. Reference to the data quality assessment procedures must be included in a coding compliance plan to establish the mechanism for determining areas of risk. Reviews will identify the need for further education and increased monitoring for those areas where either coding variances or documentation deficiencies are identified.

Specific and detailed coding guidelines that cover the reporting of typical services provided by a facility or organization create tools for data consistency and reliability by ensuring that all coders interpret clinical documentation and apply coding principles in the same manner. The appropriate medical staff committee should give final approval of any coding guidelines that involve clinical criteria to assure appropriateness and physician consensus on the process.

The format is most useful when organized by patient or service type and easily referenced by using a table of contents. If the facility-specific guidelines are maintained electronically, they should be searchable by key terms. Placing the coding guidelines on a facility Intranet or internal computer network is a very efficient way to ensure their use and it also enables timely and efficient updating and distribution. Inclusion of references to or live links should be provided to supporting documents such as Uniform Hospital Discharge Data Sets or other regulatory requirements outlining reporting procedures or code assignments.

Prepared by

AHIMA's Coding Practice Team and reviewed by the Coding Policy and Strategy Committee and the Society for Clinical Coding Data Quality Committee

Appendix C

AHIMA Practice Brief: Developing a Physician Query Process

Principles of Medical Record Documentation

Medical record documentation is used for a multitude of purposes, including:

- serving as a means of communication between the physician and the other members of the healthcare team providing care to the patient

- serving as a basis for evaluating the adequacy and appropriateness of patient care

- providing data to support insurance claims

- assisting in protecting the legal interests of patients, healthcare professionals, and healthcare facilities

- providing clinical data for research and education

To support these various uses, it is imperative that medical record documentation be complete, accurate, and timely. Facilities are expected to comply with a number of standards regarding medical record completion and content promulgated by multiple regulatory agencies.

Joint Commission on Accreditation of Healthcare Organizations

The Joint Commission's *2000 Hospital Accreditation Standards* state, "the medical record contains sufficient information to identify the patient, support the diagnosis, justify the treatment, document the course and results, and promote continuity among health care providers" (IM.7.2).[1] The Joint Commission Standards also state, "medical record data and information are managed in a timely manner" (IM.7.6).

Timely entries are essential if a medical record is to be useful in a patient's care. A complete medical record is also important when a patient is discharged, because information in the record may be needed for clinical, legal, or performance improvement purposes. The Joint Commission requires hospitals to have policy and procedures on the timely entry of all significant clinical

Source: Prophet, Sue. 2001 (October). Practice brief: Developing a physician query process. *Journal of American Health Information Management Association* 72(9):88I–M.

information into the patient's medical record, and they do not consider a medical record complete until all final diagnoses and complications are recorded without the use of symbols or abbreviations.

Joint Commission standards also require medical records to be reviewed on an ongoing basis for completeness of timeliness of information, and action is taken to improve the quality and timeliness of documentation that affects patient care (IM.7.10). This review must address the presence, timeliness, legibility, and authentication of the final diagnoses and conclusions at termination of hospitalization.

Medicare

The Medicare Conditions of Participation require medical records to be accurately written, promptly completed, properly filed and retained, and accessible.[2] Records must document, as appropriate, complications, hospital-acquired infections, and unfavorable reactions to drugs and anesthesia. The conditions also stipulate that all records must document the final diagnosis with completion of medical records within 30 days following discharge.

Relationship Between Coding and Documentation

Complete and accurate diagnostic and procedural coded data must be available, in a timely manner, in order to:

- improve the quality and effectiveness of patient care

- ensure equitable healthcare reimbursement

- expand the body of medical knowledge

- make appropriate decisions regarding healthcare policies, delivery systems, funding, expansion, and education

- monitor resource utilization

- permit identification and resolution of medical errors

- improve clinical decision making

- facilitate tracking of fraud and abuse

- permit valid clinical research, epidemiological studies, outcomes and statistical analyses, and provider profiling

- provide comparative data to consumers regarding costs and outcomes, average charges, and outcomes by procedure

Physician documentation is the cornerstone of accurate coding. Therefore, assuring the accuracy of coded data is a shared responsibility between coding professionals and physicians. Accurate diagnostic and procedural coded data originate from collaboration between physicians, who have a clinical background, and coding professionals, who have an understanding of classification systems.

Expectations of Physicians

Physicians are expected to provide complete, accurate, timely, and legible documentation of pertinent facts and observations about an individual's health history, including past and present illnesses, tests, treatments, and outcomes. Medical record entries should be documented at the time service is provided. Medical record entries should be authenticated. If subsequent additions to documentation are needed, they should be identified as such and dated. (Often these expectations are included in the medical staff or house staff rules and regulations.) Medical record documentation should:

- address the clinical significance of abnormal test results

- support the intensity of patient evaluation and treatment and describe the thought processes and complexity of decision making

- include all diagnostic and therapeutic procedures, treatments, and tests performed, in addition to their results

- include any changes in the patient's condition, including psychosocial and physical symptoms

- include all conditions that coexist at the time of admission, that subsequently develop, or that affect the treatment received and the length of stay. This encompasses all conditions that affect patient care in terms of requiring clinical evaluation, therapeutic treatment, diagnostic procedures, extended length of hospital stay, or increased nursing care and monitoring[3]

- be updated as necessary to reflect all diagnoses relevant to the care or services provided

- be consistent and discuss and reconcile any discrepancies (this reconciliation should be documented in the medical record)

- be legible and written in ink, typewritten, or electronically signed, stored, and printed

Expectations of Coding Professionals

The AHIMA Code of Ethics sets forth ethical principles for the HIM profession. HIM professionals are responsible for maintaining and promoting ethical practices. This Code of Ethics states, in part: "Health information management professionals promote high standards for health information management practice, education, and research." Another standard in this code states, "Health information management professionals strive to provide accurate and timely information." Data accuracy and integrity are fundamental values of HIM that are advanced by:

- employing practices that produce complete, accurate, and timely information to meet the health and related needs of individuals

- following the guidelines set forth in the organization's compliance plan for reporting improper preparation, alteration, or suppression of information or data by others

- not participating in any improper preparation, alteration, or suppression of health record information or other organization data

A conscientious goal for coding and maintaining a quality database is accurate clinical and statistical data. AHIMA's Standards of Ethical Coding were developed to guide coding professionals in this process. As stated in the standards, coding professionals are expected to support the importance of accurate, complete, and consistent coding practices for the production of quality healthcare data. These standards also indicate that coding professionals should only assign and report codes that are clearly and consistently supported by physician documentation in the medical record. It is the responsibility of coding professionals to assess physician documentation to assure that it supports the diagnosis and procedure codes reported on claims. Dialogue between coding professionals and clinicians is encouraged, because it improves coding professionals' clinical knowledge and educates the physicians on documentation practice issues. AHIMA's Standards of Ethical Coding state that coding professionals are expected to consult physicians for clarification and additional documentation prior to code assignment when there is conflicting or ambiguous data in the health record. Coding professionals should also assist and educate physicians by advocating proper documentation practices, further specificity, and resequencing or inclusion of diagnoses or procedures when needed to more accurately reflect the acuity, severity, and the occurrence of events. It is recommended that coding be performed by credentialed HIM professionals.[4] It is inappropriate for coding professionals to misrepresent the patient's clinical picture through incorrect coding or add diagnoses or procedures unsupported by the documentation to maximize reimbursement or meet insurance policy coverage requirements. Coding professionals should not change codes or the narratives of codes on the billing abstract so that meanings are misrepresented. Diagnoses or procedures should not be inappropriately included or excluded, because payment or insurance policy coverage requirements will be affected. When individual payer policies conflict with official coding rules and guidelines, these policies should be obtained in writing whenever possible. Reasonable efforts should be made to educate the payer on proper coding practices in order to influence a change in the payer's policy.

Proper Use of Physician Queries

The process of querying physicians is an effective and, in today's healthcare environment, necessary mechanism for improving the quality of coding and medical record documentation and capturing complete clinical data. Query forms have become an accepted tool for communicating with physicians on documentation issues influencing proper code assignment. Query forms should be used in a judicious and appropriate manner. They must be used as a communication tool to improve the accuracy of code assignment and the quality of physician documentation, not to inappropriately maximize reimbursement. The query process should be guided by AHIMA's Standards of Ethical Coding and the official coding guidelines. An inappropriate query—such as a form that is poorly constructed or asks leading questions—or overuse of the query process can result in quality-of-care, legal, and ethical concerns.

The Query Process

The goal of the query process should be to improve physician documentation and coding professionals' understanding of the unique clinical situation, not to improve reimbursement. Each facility should establish a policy and procedure for obtaining physician clarification of documentation that affects code assignment. The process of querying physicians must be a patient-specific process, not a general process. Asking "blanket" questions is not appropriate. Policies regarding the circumstances when physicians will be queried should be designed to promote timely, complete, and accurate coding and documentation. Physicians should not be asked to provide clarification of their medical record documentation without the opportunity to access the patient's medical record. Each facility also needs to determine if physicians will be queried concurrently (during the patient's hospitalization) or after discharge. Both methods are acceptable. Querying physicians concurrently allows the documentation deficiency to be corrected while the patient is still in-house and can positively influence patient care. The policy and procedure should stipulate who is authorized to contact the physician for clarifications regarding a coding issue. Coding professionals should be allowed to contact physicians directly for clarification, rather than limiting this responsibility to supervisory personnel or a designated individual. The facility may wish to use a designated physician liaison to resolve conflicts between physicians and coding professionals. The appropriate use of the physician liaison should be described in the facility's policy and procedures.

Query Format

Each facility should develop a standard format for the query form. No "sticky notes" or scratch paper should be allowed. Each facility should develop a standard design and format for physician queries to ensure clear, consistent, appropriate queries. The query form should:

- be clearly and concisely written
- contain precise language
- present the facts from the medical record and identify why clarification is needed
- present the scenario and state a question that asks the physician to make a clinical interpretation of a given diagnosis or condition based on treatment, evaluation, monitoring, and/or services provided. "Open-ended" questions that allow the physician to document the specific diagnosis are preferable to multiple-choice questions or questions requiring only a "yes" or "no" response. Queries that appear to lead the physician to provide a particular response could lead to allegations of inappropriate upcoding
- be phrased such that the physician is allowed to specify the correct diagnosis. It should not indicate the financial impact of the response to the query. The form should not be designed so that all that is required is a physician signature
- include:
  —patient name
  —admission date
  —medical record number
  —name and contact information (phone number and e-mail address) of the coding professional
  —specific question and rationale (that is, relevant documentation or clinical findings)
  —place for physician to document his or her response
  —place for the physician to sign and date his or her response

The query forms should not:

- "lead" the physician
- sound presumptive, directing, prodding, probing, or as though the physician is being led to make an assumption

- ask questions that can be responded to in a "yes" or "no" fashion
- indicate the financial impact of the response to the query
- be designed so that all that is required is a physician signature

When Is a Query Appropriate?

Physicians should be queried whenever there is conflicting, ambiguous, or incomplete information in the medical record regarding any significant reportable condition or procedure. Querying the physician only when reimbursement is affected will skew national healthcare data and might lead to allegations of upcoding.

Every discrepancy or issue not addressed in the physician documentation should not necessarily result in the physician being queried. Each facility needs to develop policies and procedures regarding the clinical conditions and documentation situations warranting a request for physician clarification. For example, insignificant or irrelevant findings may not warrant querying the physician regarding the assignment of an additional diagnosis code. Also, if the maximum number of codes that can be entered in the hospital information system has already been assigned, the facility may decide that it is not necessary to query the physician regarding an additional code. Facilities need to balance the value of marginal data being collected against the administrative burden of obtaining the additional documentation.

Members of the medical staff in consultation with coding professionals should develop the specific clinical criteria for a valid query. The specific clinical documentation that must be present in the patient's record to generate a query should be described. For example, anemia, septicemia, and respiratory failure are conditions that often require physician clarification. The medical staff can assist the coding staff in determining when it would be appropriate to query a physician regarding the reporting of these conditions by describing the specific clinical indications in the medical record documentation that raise the possibility that the condition in question may be present.

When Is a Query Not Necessary?

Queries are not necessary if a physician involved in the care and treatment of the patient, including consulting physicians, has documented a diagnosis and there is no conflicting documentation from another physician. Medical record documentation from any physician involved in the care and treatment of the patient, including documentation by consulting physicians, is appropriate for the basis of code assignment. If documentation from different physicians conflicts, seek clarification from the attending physician, as he or she is ultimately responsible for the final diagnosis.

Queries are also not necessary when a physician has documented a final diagnosis and clinical indicator—such as test results—do not appear to support this diagnosis. While coding professionals are expected to advocate complete and accurate physician documentation and to collaborate with physicians to realize this goal, they are not expected to challenge the physician's medical judgment in establishing the patient's diagnosis. However, because a discrepancy between clinical findings and a final diagnosis is a clinical issue, a facility may choose to establish a policy that the physician will be queried in these instances.

Documentation of Query Response

The physician's response to the query must be documented in the patient's medical record. Each facility must develop a policy regarding the specific process for incorporating this additional documentation in the medical record. For example, this policy might stipulate that the physician is required to add the additional information to the body of the medical record. As an alternative, a form, such as a medical record "progress note" form, might be attached to the query form and the attachment is then filed in the medical record. However, another alternative is to file the query form itself in the permanent medical record. Any documentation obtained post-discharge must be included in the discharge summary or identified as a late entry or addendum.

Any decision to file this form in the medical record should involve the advice of the facility's corporate compliance officer and legal counsel, due to potential compliance and legal risks related to incorporating the actual query form into the permanent medical record (such as its potential use as evidence of poor documentation in an audit, investigation, or malpractice suit, risks related to naming a nonclinician in the medical record, or quality of care concerns if the physician response on a query form is not clearly supported by the rest of the medical record documentation).

If the query form will serve as the only documentation of the physician's clarification, the use of "open-ended" questions (that require the physician to specifically document the additional information) are preferable to multiple choice questions or the use of questions requiring only a "yes" or "no" answer. The query form would need to be approved by the medical staff/medical records committee before implementation of a policy allowing this form to be maintained in the medical record. Also keep in mind that the Joint Commission hospital accreditation standards stipulate that only authorized individuals may make entries in medical records (IM.7.1.1). Therefore, the facility needs to consider modifying the medical staff bylaws to specify coding professionals as individuals authorized to make medical record entries prior to allowing query forms to become a permanent part of the medical record.

Auditing, Monitoring, and Corrective Action

Ideally, complete and accurate physician documentation should occur at the time care is rendered. The need for a query form results from incomplete, conflicting, or ambiguous documentation, which is an indication of poor documentation. Therefore, query form usage should be the exception rather than the norm. If physicians are being queried frequently, facility management or an appropriate medical staff committee should investigate the reasons why.

A periodic review of the query practice should include a determination of what percentage of the query forms are eliciting negative and positive responses from the physicians. A high negative response rate may be an indication that the coding staff are not using the query process judiciously and are being overzealous.

A high positive response rate may indicate that there are widespread poor documentation habits that need to be addressed. It may also indicate that the absence of certain reports (for example, discharge summary, operative report) at the time of coding is forcing the coding staff to query the physicians to obtain the information they need for proper coding.

If this is the case, the facility may wish to reconsider its policy regarding the availability of certain reports prior to coding. Waiting for these reports may make more sense in terms of turnaround time and productivity rather than finding it necessary to frequently query the physicians. The question of why final diagnoses are not available at the time of discharge may arise at the time of an audit, review by the peer review organization, or investigation.

The use of query forms should also be monitored for patterns, and any identified patterns should be used to educate physicians on improving their documentation at the point of care. If a pattern is identified, such as a particular physician or diagnosis, appropriate steps should be taken to correct the problem so the necessary documentation is present prior to coding in the future and the need to query this physician, or to query physicians regarding a particular diagnosis, is reduced. Corrective action might include targeted education for one physician or education for the entire medical staff on the proper documentation necessary for accurate code assignment.

Patterns of poor documentation that have not been addressed through education or other corrective action are signs of an ineffective compliance program. The Department of Health and Human Services Office of Inspector General has noted in its Compliance Program Guidance for Hospitals that "accurate coding depends upon the quality of completeness of the physician's documentation" and "active staff physician participation in educational programs focusing on coding and documentation should be emphasized by the hospital."[5]

The format of the queries should also be monitored on a regular basis to ensure that they are not inappropriately leading the physician to provide a particular response. Inappropriately written queries should be used to educate the coding staff on a properly written query. Patterns of inappropriately written queries should be referred to the corporate compliance officer.

Prepared by

Sue Prophet, RHIA, CCS

Acknowledgments

AHIMA Advocacy and Policy Task Force
AHIMA's Coding Practice Team
AHIMA Coding Policy and Strategy Committee
AHIMA Society for Clinical Coding
Dan Rode, MBA, FHFMA

Notes

1. Joint Commission on Accreditation of Healthcare Organizations. *Comprehensive Accreditation Manual for Hospitals: The Official Handbook.* Oakbrook Terrace, IL: Joint Commission, 2000.

2. Health Care Financing Administration, Department of Health and Human Services. "Conditions of Participation for Hospitals." Code of Federal Regulations, 2000. 42 CFR, Chapter IV, Part 482.

3. *Official ICD-9-CM Guidelines for Coding and Reporting* developed and approved by the American Hospital Association, American Health Information Management Association, Health Care Financing Administration, and the National Center for Health Statistics.

4. AHIMA is the professional organization responsible for issuing several credentials in health information management: Registered Health Information Administrator (RHIA), Registered Health Information Technician (RHIT), Certified Coding Specialist (CCS), and Certified Coding Specialist–Physician-based (CCS-P).

5. Office of Inspector General, Department of Health and Human Services. "Compliance Program Guidance for Hospitals." Washington, DC: Office of Inspector General, 1998.

References

AHIMA Code of Ethics, 1998.

AHIMA Standards of Ethical Coding, 1999.

AHIMA Coding Policy and Strategy Committee. "Practice Brief: Data Quality." *Journal of AHIMA* 67, no. 2 (1996).

Clinical Documentation Query for Physician Progress Note

Patient Name: _____ Physician Queried:_____

MR# _____ Query Date: _____

The Clinical Documentation Coordinator has reviewed the medical record in order to ensure that the principal diagnosis and all secondary diagnoses are accurately documented in the medical record. The record needs to reflect the severity of illness and expected risk of mortality for the patient.

*It appears that additional clinical documentation may be necessary. Please review the query/queries below. **If you agree with the documentation query, please document the diagnosis/diagnoses in the Physician Progress Notes.***

_____

_____

_____

_____

_____

_____

_____

_____

_____

_____

_____

_____

_____

_____

_____

_____

_____

_____

Thank you in advance for reviewing this record and documenting additional definitive diagnosis/diagnoses.

For questions, please contact: _____ *phone* _____

If you agree with the documentation query please initial here and check the appropriate physician box. _____ • **Attending Physician** • **Resident**	**If you disagree with the query please specify on this sheet why the query was not appropriate and initial here.** _____

• **ALL RESPONSES AND NO RESPONSES WILL BE REVIEWED BY THE DIVISION CHIEFS**

DO NOT DISCARD—SEND WITH THE MEDICAL RECORD AT DISCHARGE

Source: Vanderbilt University Medical Center.

Appendix D

Data Quality: The Impact on Healthcare and HIM

Executive Summary

Understanding the major elements in setting up and maintaining a vigorous data quality program across multiple hospital departments is a critical health information management skill. While accurate data is the heart of a good decision support system, consistent processes and education of key data "consumers" are also integral to success.

Key Words

Charge Description Master (CDM)

Data Quality/Integrity

Data Quality Manager (DQM)

Information Integrity Officers (IIC)

Master Patient Index (MPI)

Office of the Inspector General (OIG)

Uniform Hospital Discharge Data Set (UHDDS)

Introduction

Data quality or integrity can be defined as the assurance of the accuracy and timeliness of information. Data integrity is a critical component of any health information system. As automation continues to increase with the development and evolution of the electronic medical record (EMR), the emphasis on the role of data quality managers and the need for a rigorous data quality monitoring program increases. Processes must be put into place to encourage quality collection of data from the beginning of the patient care process, as well as to continually monitor and improve the data throughout its use until the patient is discharged.

Source: Grzybowski, Darice M. 2003 (October). *Proceedings from AHIMA's 75th Anniversary National Convention and Exhibit Proceedings.* Chicago: AHIMA.

Importance of Data Quality

Each data element collected during the patient care process becomes the building block for good information. The information that is generated in the process of patient care can be clinical, financial, or demographic. Common uses of this data include:

- Patient care,

- Tracking performance improvement and outcomes measurements,

- Negotiating managed care and other financial contracts,

- Business functions such as planning, marketing, and budgeting,

- Clinical research,

- Proof of legal compliance and reduced liability,

- Accurate billing and reimbursement (the revenue cycle), and

- Other decision support applications.

Quality data is derived directly from quality documentation. Data provided to a health-care facility generally begins with a physician order. At the point when the initial admitting diagnosis and orders are provided, the patient's record begins, along with the assignment of a medical record and/or account number for each visit. According to recent information from Zimmerman and Associates,[1] an industry consulting firm, data errors are made at the point of patient registration at a rate of between 7 and 22 percent. From that moment on, the value of the data is only as good as the continued collection and documentation of that information throughout the patient care process until final bill payment. The cost of re-billing a claim that contains errors has been estimated anywhere between $27 and $100 per claim. If the average error rate on registrations is 14.5 percent, and the average re-bill cost is $63.50, with the average volume of daily registrations (inpatient and outpatient) at about 600 daily cases, the cost of re-billing could amount to more than $5,000 a day.

Good data has value that impacts every aspect of healthcare—case management, Joint Commission accreditation (Core Measures), physician credentialing, accounts receivable collections, and much more. Since the attack on September 11, there has been a greater awareness in the healthcare industry of the impact and use of quality coded data to support public health alerts and as an early warning system of possible bioterrorism attacks.

How Data Is Collected

Understanding where and how data is generated is essential to establishing a true data quality program. There are six major areas within a hospital where data is created and collected. The data created by each area forms the core of a comprehensive data repository.

1. The first, and most important, is the master patient index (MPI). The MPI captures basic patient identification and demographic data and serves as an index to a patient's entire visit history. It is considered a legal document and is usually required to be maintained permanently.

2. The second data collection point is charge line items that are generated from the charge description master (CDM). This is also referred to as the service item master

(SIM) by clinicians. Charges are selected and collected as part of the patient care process and are used for billing as well as to measure critical pathway treatment variances and patterns.

3. Clinical documentation is a form of data collection. Whether handwritten or generated as part of an order, dictated and transcribed, or electronically generated from a legacy clinical system, the data collected in the documentation process provides the key information upon which statistical data is gathered in the remainder of the healthcare process.

4. Until the completion of patient care, most of the documentation and data collected is in "raw" form and exists in what is referred to as the source document, or original point of data collection. It is at this juncture that most electronic and manual records are scanned, and professional staff review and interpret the data into codified data sets and abstracted data summaries. Sometimes, there are multiple abstracting systems and data sets used to collect this information. This process is complex, time-consuming, and critical to a hospital's ability to utilize data for any comparative or clinical research, and to process existing claims data for payment. The process of coding and abstracting generally requires very specific software designed to make this process efficient and accurate.

5. The UB-04 is generally considered *the* primary billing format for hospitals, although facilities that perform physician billing also utilize the CMS-1500 format. The UB-04 contains most elements of the uniform hospital discharge data set (UHDDS), and it is generally considered a good summary of the basics of a patient-specific visit, minus clinical values.

6. Other decision support systems and data repositories make up the last of the critical data gathering sets. Information is generally loaded into these systems from other entry points, yet these systems are commonly the final resting and access points for much of the facility's data, after other source documents and files are purged earlier.

How Data Is Monitored

Since data originates in so many different places within a healthcare facility, monitoring to ensure accurate collection is often a challenge. Implementation of policies and procedures can support this process and should include guidelines for collection of the data as well as procedures for the correction or revision of data. A data dictionary that provides a glossary of key data elements is essential and should be standardized throughout the organization. A multidisciplinary team consisting of members from HIM, patient registration, nursing, finance, patient financial services, the medical staff, and information services should be granted the oversight authority to maintain this dictionary.

Forms control is also essential. Whether manual or electronic, standardization of forms, including number control, format, design, and content, should be tightly monitored. This not only ensures better data, but also can result in large cost savings for the facility. Improving forms control also helps prepare those facilities for implementation of document imaging and workflow, which is essential to the foundation of an electronic medical record.

Edits and audits are an important part of any data monitoring system. Healthcare facilities can implement systems that provide automated checks, or institute data quality review programs such as a routine and random check on collected data against a set of standard accuracy criteria. This is also helpful for providing performance feedback to employees and can serve a dual purpose by meeting continuous quality improvement initiatives of accrediting agencies. The key is accountability among all staff for the collection of accurate and timely data.

Improving the Data

After monitoring the quality of the data, the next step is to improve the data collection process. This is often a difficult step, as behavioral change in the process of data collection is often resisted. Providing empirical data through the use of run charts and statistics that clearly note the denominator and numerator of what is being studied is a sure way to initiate action. At the same time, care must be taken not to overreact to numbers without analyzing the data. For example, a physician may claim that 20 radiology reports in a single month contained significant errors. However, upon investigation, the reports containing errors were 16 percent of the total reports transcribed that month, and the "significant" errors were primarily grammatical in nature. If a single report contained a potentially problematic clinical error, it could be argued that it may have been correctly transcribed based on the actual dictation. In-depth analysis of the data can uncover the root causes of a specific problem.

When analyzing situations that produce faulty data, attention should focus on the five Ws:

- WHO gathers the data is important. Someone with a lack of understanding of how a system works or the terminology used might create a problem due to ignorance. Often there is a lack of resources to manage the data properly—one only needs to listen to a nurse complain that he or she is there to "take care of patients," not to "worry about the census being accurate" to understand the difficulty facilities face when healthcare professionals not necessarily suited to the task of data collection are required to assume multiple roles.

- The WHAT is important. If there is not a clear understanding of the limits of what data is being collected, contamination of data can occur. A common example is collecting free-form narrative diagnosis information when a codified entry is desirable.

- WHERE data is collected is essential, as a noisy environment can lead to distraction and data entry errors.

- WHEN the data is collected is also a key issue. Concurrency is always the best policy to promote timeliness and accuracy. What good does it do for the front desk to know a patient was transferred into observation services this morning, if the location of the patient wasn't updated until after the patient was admitted as an inpatient and the family had spent a half hour roaming the halls looking for their loved one?

- Finally, WHY data is needed is also important to understand. Countless hours of wasted productivity can occur because of over-collection, over-documentation, and over-reporting. Medical record "size" has doubled and in some cases the paper chart has quadrupled in thickness with duplicative information being collected manually and electronically. The problem is magnified by poorly designed computerized output of many clinical documentation systems. With good forms control, streamlining of essential data elements saves time and dollars and produces better codified data sets in the end.

The final tip in improving data quality is to focus on one improvement effort at a time. If the goal is to reduce the incidence of duplicate medical record numbers assigned to less than

1 percent, don't stop monitoring this process until that improvement goal is met. Without rein-forcement, buy in, and accountability, the problem may return.

Challenges and Opportunities

There are several significant areas in healthcare that tend to be traps for creating repetitive problems in data quality. Four of the most common areas are described below:

- Improving Your Master Patient Index Data: Preregistering patients and creating an active account number before they arrive for admission can lead to extra census entries and "zero charge" false cases in the master patient index. Proper preregistration and collection of data is fine, but the activation of the account/visit should not occur until a patient is physically present in a facility or an actual specimen (in the case of a reference lab) is received. Entering inaccurate dates (admission, transfer, and discharge) can lead to a variety of problems, including wrong charge calculation, errors in length-of-stay calculations, and other potential issues. Do you really know your MPI? How do you register patients who are solely filling a prescription? Do you allow alias names, and how do you reconcile this with the real patient information?

- A, B, C, D, E Audits: The audit I recommend the most is an audit that is actually a validity check verifying the consistency between the data at various points in the patient care process cycle. A represents the order, B represents the results (documentation in the medical record) C, the charges that should match the test/process/treatment that was completed, D, the coding that should capture the data, and E, the data generated on the bill. All of these elements should match in content, yet surprisingly, 3M consultants conducting these audits have found that 60 percent of cases have at least one problem. Try this at your own facility and you may be amazed by what you find.

- Data Interpretation: It's surprising how different people interpret data definitions. Unfortunately, most facilities operate without a data dictionary to help standardize terms. Those organizations that have a data dictionary are still often plagued by the fact that different information systems may define the same term in a variety of ways. Try administering a quiz to the leadership in your facility: ask staff to define who the "admitting" physician is in the emergency department, what their definition of an observation patient is, when they consider the official time of surgery start to be, and what the official day of admission is for a patient who is converted to inpatient status after midnight following treatment the previous evening in the emergency department.

- Data Comparisons: For data to be used for comparative purposes, it must be normalized as much as possible, and severity-adjusted as well. Most facilities, however, don't get to that point because they still haven't addressed the basic issues of data collection. This includes deciding which database or system will be used for what purpose. It also includes deciding who is the owner of that data, from both an accurate collection and a final maintenance perspective. Certain systems are designed for more accurate reporting for specific types of abstracted data than others. While eliminating redundant and stand-alone databases is the best approach whenever possible, in some cases a financial decision support system may not be designed to adequately meet the needs of a clinical outcomes and quality management reporting system. It may be necessary to implement a system expressly designed for quality purposes. Finally, every data element in every system should have its own history and owner.

Data Quality and Compliance

The Centers for Medicare and Medicaid Services (CMS), through the Office of the Inspector General (OIG), intensified efforts to study data integrity through their fraud and abuse monitoring system established in 1996. Under the general heading of "Compliance," OIG efforts targeted correct coding, classification, documentation, and billing issues in healthcare. Noncompliance can result in extensive penalty fines for a facility and a nightmare for the organization's public relations department. The key focus in the compliance area has been looking at the relationship between documentation, coded data, and bill submission.

Recent advances in automated software help eliminate inconsistencies in these three areas. Automation has begun to redefine how systems can evaluate the data that is being captured, and allows for a greater percentage of auditing of records than ever before. Advances in the use of clinical and resource edits, combined with artificial intelligence tools and natural language processing, will expand the new technologies available to the healthcare market. The use of internal and external consultants to provide process improvement guidelines for documentation, coded data, and bill submission has also proliferated.

A Final Lesson

Data quality is a complex issue and takes dedicated tracking and resources to ensure its accuracy. The data quality cycle is very similar to the quality improvement cycle. The first step is to detect or identify where problems exist. The second step is the correction of identified problems by improving the process of collection. The third step is to prevent future problems by increasing accountability of individuals involved with data collection. It is essential that these individuals be educated as to the importance of improved data accuracy. The final step is to verify that a valid audit process for data quality is in place. Trended data is the key to documenting the quality of the data in an organization's system.

Looking to the future, the AHIMA Vision 2006 role of data quality manager[2] is now becoming a reality. In the September 2002 issue of *Medical Records Briefing,*[3] an HIM industry newsletter, the position of a data integrity specialist is described as a critical role in one hospital's operations. In the November/December 2002 issue of the *Journal of AHIMA,*[4] Linda Kloss, AHIMA executive vice president and CEO, refers to this new role for HIM professionals as an "information integrity officer" and states, "Information integrity has the potential for becoming a new discipline, a new science, even a new industry, very much like environmental science and industry, which emerged as a result of society's concerns. . . ."

Whether it is as a leader in the implementation of a data monitoring system, a database "clean up" specialist, a coding or transcription "edits" analyst, or a full-fledged data quality manager, HIM professionals can look to the future as a time to be involved, engaged, and contributing to the quality of the healthcare system and its information. Let us all champion the cause of quality healthcare data.

Endnotes

1. Zimmerman and Associates. Revenue Cycle Management Summit, Chicago, IL. (May 8, 2003).

2. Cassidy, Bonnie. "Vision 2006 Brings Data Quality Management into View." *Journal of AHIMA* Vol. 69, no. 6 (1998): 28–31.

3. *Medical Records Briefing* Vol. 17, No. 9 (September 2002): 6.

4. Kloss, Linda. "Information Integrity: Our Achilles' Heel." *Journal of AHIMA* (November/Dec 2002): 23.

Appendix E

AHIMA Practice Brief: Managing and Improving Data Quality

Complete and accurate diagnostic and procedural coded data is necessary for research, epidemiology, outcomes and statistical analyses, financial and strategic planning, reimbursement, evaluation of quality of care, and communication to support the patient's treatment.

Consistency of coding has been a major AHIMA initiative in the quest to improve data quality management in healthcare service reporting. The Association has also taken a stand on the quality of healthcare data and information.[1]

Data Quality Mandates

Adherence to industry standards and approved coding principles that generate coded data of the highest quality and consistency remains critical to the healthcare industry and the maintenance of information integrity throughout healthcare systems. HIM professionals must continue to meet the challenges of maintaining an accurate and meaningful database reflective of patient mix and resource use. As long as diagnostic and procedural codes serve as the basis for payment methodologies, the ethics of clinical coders and healthcare organization billing processes will be challenged.

Ensuring accuracy of coded data is a shared responsibility between HIM professionals, clinicians, business services staff, and information systems integrity professionals. The HIM professional has the unique responsibility of administration, oversight, analysis, and/or coding clinical data in all healthcare organizations. Care must be taken in organizational structures to ensure that oversight of the coding and data management process falls within the HIM department's responsibility area so data quality mandates are upheld and appropriate HIM principles are applied to business practices.

Clinical Collaboration

The Joint Commission and the Medicare Conditions of Participation as well as other accreditation agencies require final diagnoses and procedures to be recorded in the medical record and authenticated by the responsible practitioner. State laws also provide guidelines concerning the content of the health record as a legal document.

Source: AHIMA Coding Products and Services Team. 2003 (July/August). Practice brief: Managing and improving data quality. *Journal of American Health Information Management Association* 74(7):64A–C.

Clinical documentation primarily created by physicians is the cornerstone of accurate coding, supplemented by appropriate policies and procedures developed by facilities to meet patient care requirements. Coded data originates from the collaboration between clinicians and HIM professionals with clinical terminology, classification system, nomenclature, data analysis, and compliance policy expertise.

Thus, the need for collaboration, cooperation, and communication between clinicians and support personnel continues to grow as information gathering and storage embrace new technology. Movement of the coding process into the business processing side of a healthcare organization must not preclude access to and regular communication with clinicians.

Clinical Database Evaluation

Regulatory agencies are beginning to apply data analysis tools to monitor data quality and reliability for reimbursement appropriateness and to identify unusual claims data patterns that may indicate payment errors or health insurance fraud. Examples include the Hospital Payment Monitoring Program Tool, First Look Analysis Tool for Hospital Outlier Monitoring (FATHOM), used by Quality Improvement Organizations, and the comprehensive error rate testing (CERT) process to be used by Centers for Medicare & Medicaid Services carriers to produce national, contractor, provider type, and benefit category-specific paid claims error rates.

Ongoing evaluation of the clinical database by health information managers facilitates ethical reporting of clinical information and early identification of data accuracy problems for timely and appropriate resolution. Pattern analysis of codes is a useful tool for prevention of compliance problems by identifying and correcting clinical coding errors.

Coding errors have multiple causes, some within the control of HIM processes and others that occur outside the scope of HIM due to inadequacy of the source document or the lack of information integrity resulting from inappropriate computer programming routines or software logic.

Data Quality Management and Improvement Initiatives

The following actions are required in any successful program:

- Evaluation and trending of diagnosis and procedure code selections, the appropriateness of reimbursement group assignment, and other coded data elements such as discharge status are required. This action ensures that clinical concept validity, appropriate code sequencing, specific code use requirements, and clinical pertinence are reflected in the codes reported

- Reporting data quality review results to organizational leadership, compliance staff, and the medical staff. This stresses accountability for data quality to everyone involved and allows the root causes of inconsistency or lack of reliability of data validity to be addressed. If the source for code assignment is inadequate or invalid, the results may reflect correct coding by the coding professional, but still represent a data quality problem because the code assigned does not reflect the actual concept or event as it occurred

- Following up on and monitoring identified problems. HIM professionals must resist the temptation to overlook inadequate documentation and report codes without appropriate clinical foundation within the record just to speed up claims processing, meet a business requirement, or obtain additional reimbursement. There is an ethical duty as members of the healthcare team to educate physicians on appropriate documentation practices and maintain high standards for health information practice. Organizational structures must support these efforts by the enforcement of medical staff rules and regulations and continuous monitoring of clinical pertinence of documentation to meet both business and patient care requirements

HIM clinical data specialists who understand data quality management concepts and the relationship of clinical code assignments to reimbursement and decision support for healthcare will have important roles to play in the healthcare organizations of the future. Continuing education and career boosting specialty advancement programs are expected to be the key to job security and professional growth as automation continues to change healthcare delivery, claims processing, and compliance activities.[2]

Data Quality Recommendations

HIM coding professionals and the organizations that employ them are accountable for data quality that requires the following behaviors.

HIM professionals should:

- Adopt best practices made known in professional resources and follow the code of ethics for the profession or their specific compliance programs.[3] This guidance applies to all settings and all health plans

- Use the entire health record as part of the coding process in order to assign and report the appropriate clinical codes for the standard transactions and codes sets required for external reporting and meeting internal abstracting requirements

- Adhere to all official coding guidelines published in the HIPAA standard transactions and code sets regulation. ICD-9-CM guidelines are available for downloading at www.cdc.gov/nchs/data/icd9/icdguide.pdf. Additional official coding advice is published in the quarterly publication AHA *Coding Clinic for ICD-9-CM*. CPT guidelines are located within the CPT code books and additional information and coding advice is provided in the AMA monthly publication *CPT Assistant*. Modifications to the initial HIPAA standards for electronic transactions or adoption of additional standards are submitted first to the designated standard maintenance organization.

- Develop appropriate facility or practice-specific guidelines when available coding guidelines do not address interpretation of the source document or guide code selection in specific circumstances. Facility practice guidelines should not conflict with official coding guidelines

- Maintain a working relationship with clinicians through ongoing communication and documentation improvement programs

- Report root causes of data quality concerns when identified. Problematic issues that arise from individual physicians or groups of clinicians should be referred to medical staff leadership or the compliance office for investigation and resolution

- Query when necessary. Best practices and coding guidelines suggest that when coding professionals encounter conflicting or ambiguous documentation in a source document, the physician must be queried to confirm the appropriate code selection[4]

- Consistently seek out innovative methods to capture pertinent information required for clinical code assignment to minimize unnecessary clinician inquiries. Alternative methods of accessing information necessary for code assignment may prevent the need to wait for completion of the health record, such as electronic access to clinical reports

- Ensure that clinical code sets reported to outside agencies are fully supported by documentation within the health record and clearly reflected in diagnostic statements and procedure reports provided by a physician

- Provide the physician the opportunity to review reported diagnoses and procedures on pre- or post-claim or post-bill submission, via mechanisms such as:

  —providing a copy (via mail, fax, or electronic transmission) of the sequenced codes and their narrative descriptions, taking appropriate care to protect patient privacy and security of the information

  —placing the diagnostic and procedural listing within the record and bringing it to the physician's attention within the appropriate time frame for correction when warranted

- Create a documentation improvement program or offer educational programs concerning the relationship of health record entries and health record management to data quality, information integrity, patient outcomes, and business success of the organization

- Conduct a periodic or ongoing review of any automated billing software (chargemasters, service description masters, practice management systems, claims scrubbers, medical necessity software) used to ensure code appropriateness and validity of clinical codes

- Require a periodic or ongoing review of encounter forms or other resource tools that involve clinical code assignment to ensure validity and appropriateness

- Complete appropriate continuing education and training to keep abreast of clinical advancements in diagnosis and treatment, billing and compliance issues, regulatory requirements, and coding guideline changes, and to maintain professional credentials

HIM coding professionals and the organizations that employ them have the responsibility to not engage in, promote, or tolerate the following behaviors that adversely affect data quality. HIM professionals should not:

- Make assumptions requiring clinical judgment concerning the etiology or context of the condition under consideration for code reporting

- Misrepresent the patient's clinical picture through code assignment for diagnoses/procedures unsupported by the documentation in order to maximize reimbursement, affect insurance policy coverage, or because of other third-party payer requirements. This includes falsification of conditions to meet medical necessity requirements when the patient's condition does not support health plan coverage for the service in question or using a specific code requested by a payer when, according to official coding guidelines, a different code is mandatory

- Omit the reporting of clinical codes that represent actual clinical conditions or services but negatively affect a facility's data profile, negate health plan coverage, or lower the reimbursement potential

- Allow changing of clinical code assignments under any circumstances without consultation with the coding professional involved and the clinician whose services are being reported. Changes are allowed only with subsequent validation of the documentation supporting the need for code revision

- Fail to use the physician query process outlined by professional practice standards or required by quality improvement organizations under contract for federal and state agencies that reimburse for healthcare services

- Assign codes to an incomplete record without organizational policies in place to ensure the codes are reviewed after the records are complete. Failure to confirm the accuracy and completeness of the codes submitted for a reimbursement claim upon completion of the medical record can increase both data quality and compliance risks[5]

- Promote or tolerate the falsification of clinical documentation or misrepresentation of clinical conditions or service provided

Prepared by

AHIMA's Coding Products and Services team:
Kathy Brouch, RHIA, CCS
Susan Hull, MPH, RHIA, CCS
Karen Kostick, RHIT, CCS, CCS-P
Rita Scichilone, MHSA, RHIA, CCS, CCS-P
Mary Stanfill, RHIA, CCS, CCS-P
Ann Zeisset, RHIT, CCS, CCS-P

Acknowledgments

AHIMA Coding (SCC) Community of Practice
AHIMA Coding Policy and Strategy Committee
Sue Prophet-Bowman, RHIA, CCS

Notes

1. For details, see AHIMA's Position Statements on Consistency of Healthcare Diagnostic and Procedural Coding and on the Quality of Healthcare Data and Information at www.ahima.org/dc/positions.

2. For more information on AHIMA's specialty advancement programs, go to http://campus.ahima.org. Institutes for Healthcare Data Analytics and Clinical Data Management are planned for the 2003 AHIMA National Convention. Visit www.ahima.org/convention for more information.

3. AHIMA's Standards of Ethical Coding are available at www.ahima.org/infocenter/guidelines.

4. Prophet, Sue. "Practice Brief: Developing a Physician Query Process." *Journal of AHIMA* 72, no. 9 (2001): 88I–M.

5. More guidelines for HIM policy and procedure development are available in Health Information Management Compliance: A Model Program for Healthcare Organizations by Sue Prophet, AHIMA, 2002. Coding from incomplete records is also discussed in the AHIMA Practice Brief "Developing a Coding Compliance Document" in the July/August 2001 *Journal of AHIMA* (vol. 72, no. 7, prepared by AHIMA's Coding Practice Team).

Appendix F

Developing an Effective Compliance Audit Process

Introduction

The dictionary definition of an audit is "a methodical examination and review." To monitor is to "watch, observe, or check, especially for a special purpose." Because of a variety of reasons in the current healthcare delivery market, assessment and monitoring of information gathering and reporting processes to ensure compliance with organizational and customer needs is a critical function. This paper will discuss the structure and process of conducting audits for compliance related to coding, reimbursement, and related documentation issues.

Background

The Payment Error Protection Program (PEPP) has resulted in a number of excellent manuals and structures for coding and reimbursement evaluation. HIM professionals can look to this resource prepared by the Peer Review Organizations (PROs) under contract with government agencies for reliable means to improve processes and minimize risk of noncompliance. The first time an audit or review process is undertaken it can be more resource intensive than subsequent review activities. A first-time look at any process is generally referred to as a "baseline assessment." It is impossible to initiate performance improvement until it is known where most problems occur. Areas for investigation must be determined, processes must be developed and documented, personnel must be identified to conduct the audit, and the audit must be performed. Baseline audits demand that a wider net be cast to ensure important deficiencies are recognized. Unidentified coding problems translate into reimbursement not received or potential liability for compliance problems. To be sure there are no surprises, the first audit must be comprehensive. Subsequent audits will be much less time-consuming because processes will have already been established, and it will be clear which areas do not require focused attention or additional review resources and time.

Audit Strategy

Subsequent audits will start the monitoring and evaluation process. Frequency of review is facility specific, and may depend on who is reviewing the information and what action will

Source: Scichilone, Rita. 2001 (October). *AHIMA National Convention Proceedings.* Chicago: AHIMA.

be taken from the results. Assessments should be conducted at regular intervals (monthly, quarterly, semiannually, annually), with the results used to monitor the effectiveness of the compliance program.

Reviews performed subsequent to the baseline measurement seek answers to the following questions:

1. For problem areas, did improvement occur since the last review?

2. For nonproblem areas, was the initial baseline level maintained, or did significant deviations occur?

3. Does any result of review require immediate referral to the compliance office for investigation of noncompliance that involves overpayments or fraudulent activity?

4. Are there any findings that require immediate referral to the business services unit or clinical department management for underreporting or missed charges?

Some organizations choose to review coding accuracy and conduct claims review separately. Coding accuracy requires individual record assessment, while some aspects of claims review are based on aggregate data analysis. Any coding assessment should include verification that the codes selected for the case are the same codes reported for any external purpose, such as reimbursement from a third party.

Section I: Coding Assessment

Code assignment review should be performed to ensure that coding is being done in compliance with coding rules and official guidelines. The baseline audit should be extensive enough to establish baseline performance (coding accuracy) in distinct areas considered to be important (e.g., settings, departments, and types of coding). As stated previously, subsequent audits, which may be smaller in scope, should be performed at regular intervals to compare the current accuracy level with the baseline accuracy level. More frequent audits may be performed in areas identified as requiring improvement. Coding audits will generally involve reviewing a sample of the population as opposed to auditing all claims. A coding audit compares the clinical documentation to the codes assigned and evaluates whether all possible codes were reported, whether they were correct, whether the documentation is inadequate for complete coding, or whether coding principles were not followed. In addition, it includes a tracking of the codes assigned on the resulting claim form to make sure the information is accurate and complete.

Selecting an Approach to a Coding Audit

A variety of means are useful to structure and approach the assessment of coding accuracy. The first step is to establish when during the coding or billing process you wish to conduct the review. Reviews may be conducted prior to billing, or after billing has occurred and payment has been received. There are advantages and disadvantages to each approach. The next step is to establish the approach you will use for selecting cases for review. Every coding staff member should have records included in the sample, and if physician documentation is under scrutiny, each physician should also have records in the sample for at least the baseline review. Once documentation adequacy has been established, this can be suspended. Most facilities review this in a cyclic fashion and make the results available at the time of medical staff reappointment or performance evaluation for employed physicians. Reviewing adequacy of documentation at the same time a coding assessment is performed is one way of keeping the process efficient and avoiding duplication of effort in pulling records and conducting review.

It is also recommended that particular areas identified as problematic are reviewed. This will be based on past audit results or on the current OIG Workplan1 that identifies high-risk areas. By doing both, you should not miss persistent coding errors in low-risk areas or errors in areas that are known to be problematic in other facilities and that represent significant risk of external review and subsequent compliance problems.

Typical Facility Coding Audit Approaches

- A facility performs quarterly retrospective coding reviews as part of its quality improvement plan. Records from each coding staff member are selected randomly for all payers. The Data Quality Coordinator performs the review by selecting 10 records for each person. Coding errors are discussed with the persons responsible and are trended to track future improvement and suggest training needs. Cases with errors that affect reimbursement are referred to the business office for rebilling when appropriate.

- A facility monitors claims containing selected DRGs and APCs that have been identified as problematic prior to billing. Any revisions are made prior to billing, thus allowing the hospital to be paid correctly the first time. This reduces the amount of rebilling and minimizes the risk of external agency focused review. The population for sample selection is limited to payers that use the reimbursement system under review.

- A facility conducts studies of remittance advices received by the billing office for trends and patterns that involve coding issues. The facility looked for inconsistencies between the DRGs assigned by the hospital coders and what was paid by the Fiscal Intermediary or insurance plan. Rebills are submitted as appropriate within the required time frame. The facility quantifies underpayments and overpayments, as well as denials. These results are logged over time to identify problem areas. Summary information is provided to the compliance committee.

- A facility conducts monthly coding accuracy reviews by using the manager of clinical data as the auditor. Samples of each coding staff member's work are pulled from all patient types—inpatient acute care, outpatient surgery, outpatient ancillary, endoscopy, emergency department, observation, and skilled care. UB-92s are pulled to make sure codes are transferring correctly. Errors are reviewed at a coding staff meeting where at least one educational topic is presented to improve skills in coding and record analysis. Each quarter, an external consulting firm conducts an independent coding review by using the same population. The consulting group also provides an in-service in conjunction with their report on areas of concern or new topics requiring special knowledge or application of unfamiliar coding guidelines.

- In addition to auditing coding accuracy, you should also review adequacy and completeness of physician medical record documentation to support optimal coding. Some facilities make this part of the medical record review function and review not only for adequacy to support code selection and justify billing but also for application of clinical pertinence criteria defined by medical staff. Records that fail the screens are referred to committee for peer review and medical staff follow-up. Documentation inadequacies for coding purposes are trended, and educational programs are provided to improve processes. For example, a hospital may choose to monitor the presence or absence of final diagnoses on the record at the time of discharge, according to medical staff rules and regulations. Another indicator may be to measure the inclusion of complications and comorbidities in the diagnostic statements or the persistent need for clarification from the coding staff because of ambiguous documentation.

Establishing Who Will Conduct the Reviews

Each facility must establish the person(s) responsible for performing the coding audits. This should begin with deciding whether to use internal or external resources. Objectivity demands that someone independent of the actual coding function conduct the reviews. Coder-to-coder peer review is effective only when the identity of the coder is concealed. It can also hide inappropriate coding practices that are universally applied even though they are incorrect. Perhaps a workshop presenter gave questionable advice or a previous supervisor instructed the coders to apply a certain interpretation of coding rules. This would not be picked up until an objective review was undertaken by a disinterested party.

The designated reviewers must all have coding expertise and credible training background. Some facilities choose to use a panel of auditors, with each providing expertise in a particular area or healthcare setting. For example, one auditor specializes in CPT coding and another specializes in ICD-9-CM coding; others may fully understand physician professional fee reporting or home health data sets or skilled nursing requirements.

A physician advisor should be available to field clinical questions or questions about the application of clinical pertinence criteria or documentation adequacy.

Documenting the Process

As with all compliance activities, it is important to develop detailed written policy and procedures for conducting audits and maintaining the results. As appropriate, the policy should identify when and how audits should be performed, what forms and criteria are used in the review process, and what is done with the results. Some compliance plans require all coding audits to be performed under the direction of legal counsel to qualify for the attorney-client privilege, work-product immunity, or other protections.

Establishing a Review Plan

The written audit plan should be in force for a specified period and reviewed at the end of its life. A written audit plan should contain at least the following elements:

1. A discussion of the established frequency for performing the audit.

2. A discussion of the established period covered by each audit.

3. A description of the population eligible for review should be specified in the audit plan, if the audit processing is ongoing and selected departments or patient types are reviewed in rotation.

4. An explanation of how the sample size will be determined, which will depend on the type of audit being conducted. Various resources provide recommendations for various types of samples; for example, a routine review is suggested to sample five percent or 30 records, whichever number is greater. A discussion of the established

sample design, in most cases a simple random sample, is sufficient, though the source of the random numbers must be documented if used for self-disclosure. For self-disclosure, the OIG recommends the use of its Office of Audit Services Statistical Sampling Software, also known as RAT-STATS (currently available free of charge through the Internet at www.hhs.gov/progorg/oas/ratstat.html). *A Guide to Auditing Health Care Billing Practices,* published by Atlantic Information Services, Inc.,[2] also contains a good sample form for the documentation of a sample selection plan, among other tools.

5. A description of the indicators (see the next section of this paper for more details).

6. A description of the planned analysis techniques.

Defining Indicators

Appropriate indicators must be defined to measure accuracy of code reporting in a consistent and fair process. One type of indicator will be the coding error rate. This must be defined by the number of records with coding errors, as compared with the number of records without coding errors. Some facilities also collect data in greater detail by comparing the number and accuracy of the codes assigned to the omissions or incorrect code assignment. This is more complicated to administer but may be more meaningful depending on what analysis is needed.

Two types of error rate categories are recommended: errors that affect reimbursement by causing a grouping error or fee-schedule payment error, and errors that do not affect reimbursement. Both are important, since they affect the reliability of data in many systems, not just the payment process. Reimbursement errors are critical because they increase risk of fraud or abuse allegations and can trigger overpayments that must be returned and impact the financial health of the organization. In developing the coding compliance program, standards for coding accuracy are clearly stated. In a perfect world, standards will be 100 percent accuracy for all coders, but each organization must consider the degree of risk associated with errors and decide for itself the level of accuracy that must be maintained. If you expect 100 percent accuracy in code assignment, you must find a way to produce 100 percent adequacy and completeness in physician documentation. Asking a coding professional to identify all reportable procedures from an incomplete record and then attributing errors to that person after review of a completed record is not fair. A defined indicator will allow you to evaluate compliance with coding accuracy standards and benchmarks. Other common indicators include areas such as accuracy of grouping assignment, selection of the principal diagnosis for inpatients, and correct selection of the discharge status.

After completion of the baseline audit, the facility should have identified problems or opportunities for improvement in the coding process. The next step is to define indicators that will show how the coding process and outcome is expected to improve by the next audit. For example, after a comprehensive training program concerning correct coding of spinal fusion procedures, you may expect the percentage of certain DRGs to decrease. Another result might be an expectation that the number of FI rejections for a particular reason will decrease or maybe the expectation is to show an increase in the case mix index (CMI). A selected indicator could be a quantitative measure of these processes that can be measured over time, such as a percentage of discharges with FI rejections or the ratio of one DRG to another in Medicare or other defined financial classes that show DRG payment impact. Sampling protocols may be used to determine when additional record review may be needed in vulnerable areas. Often, serious problems can be prevented if an effective monitoring process is in place to catch coding aberrations early and allow immediate intervention.

Designing Reports, Compiling Results, and Effecting Change

Report formats for tracking and analyzing coding audit results must be customized to the audience. Reports should allow tracking overall coding accuracy and the accuracy of individual employees. They should also allow monitoring of those areas you have determined to be problematic so improvement or backsliding is evident and can be addressed. In general, charts and graphs are worth 10 text descriptions, especially with management-level users or physicians. Any employee or physician results should be encrypted for public display, with details available for authorized and appropriate personnel.

Using Audit Results

The results of coding assessments and any corrective action implemented as a result should be summarized and submitted to the compliance officer for consideration and maintenance. Legal counsel should be consulted in deciding how results will be documented and who is authorized access to the reports.

Section II: Claims Auditing

Because the coding process and the billing process for third-party reimbursement are so integrated and dependent on each other, claims audits should be performed to ensure that claims are processed in accordance with required healthcare program and billing regulations.

Electronic databases of paid claims enable an organization to access the entire universe of their claims in aggregate. Compare this to coding audits for which it is practical to review only samples of the population. Any facility without an electronic database should consider reviewing each claim process along with the coding review and perhaps selecting additional cases purely for claims processing review.

Selecting an Approach to a Claims Audit

Auditing of claims can be approached from three different perspectives. Use of reimbursement methods such as the DRG and APC can provide frequency reports, so a "big picture" view can be created about the nature of the services being reported. Some claims reviews include an audit to determine completeness of medical record documentation in supporting the services billed. Finally, any claims review process must consider the codes selected by the coding staff or physician and include those dropped in the charge description master, as compared with the codes submitted to the FI or carrier to ensure that they are exactly the same.

The second and third perspectives are actually extensions of the coding audit, and the same guidelines provided in the previous section apply to the claims review process. Some facilities choose to separate the reviews, since they focus on different objectives, while others choose to combine the reviews to minimize pulling of records and overlapping tasks. To meet market demand, vendors have created software programs that profile facilities' claims data and/or search for upcoding or trends requiring further study. Some of these programs may be very valuable in helping you audit because of the amount of analysis they can provide, but exercise caution in their selection. The OIG recently tested software designed to detect upcoding and achieved only modest success.[3] The analyses proposed in this section are simple to conduct if a facility can perform basic queries of their database systems and do not require purchase of additional software.

Establishing Who Will Conduct Claims Audits

As with the coding reviews, it is important to establish who will perform the audits and how the review process interacts with the coding assessment process. Each facility needs to evaluate whether the organization has the internal resources to perform the work or if an auditing firm with the required expertise should be hired. Both options have advantages, and a blend of the two strategies is preferred. The use of internal staff should represent cost-savings over hiring an outside contractor. For billing reviews, additional expertise is required to identify missed charges or billing process errors, and some coding experts may not have this knowledge without specific training or experience. An experienced auditing firm can bring knowledge of other clients' situations to identify risk areas. Ideally, a facility would acquaint itself with its data and data systems before bringing in an outside contractor. Some health systems employ internal auditors that fill this role. They must work closely with the HIM or coding personnel in a facility to ensure optimal review results.

Documenting the Process of Claims Audits

As with the coding assessment, a detailed policy and procedure for conducting the audits is prepared. The policy should identify when and how audits should be conducted and the circumstances of working under the direction of legal counsel to maintain legal protection under the attorney-client or work-product privileges. Report formats are developed that will be used to compile results to meet the objectives of a claims-processing review.

Establishing the Audit Plan

The audit plan should include:

- Audit frequency
- Time period
- Review population
- Sample size and sample design (if using sampling)
- Indicators
- Indicator specifications
- Time frames
- Comparative data or benchmarks
- Analysis techniques

Identifying the Necessary Personnel for Claims Audits

A team of individuals from various departments may be assembled to assist with developing claims-auditing procedures. Generally, a project of this scope requires individuals from various disciplines throughout the organization because of the widespread use of chargemasters and/or charge tickets for many items. HIM staff will be called on to identify important coding issues and develop coding accuracy and/or grouping assignment indicators, while billing department staff will be called on to guide the selection of appropriate claims and their data sources. When working with aggregate data, information services staff will be helpful in creating automated tools and programs for retrieving all the necessary data.

The compliance officer and the compliance committee should oversee the process and provide input into how it is conducted and who should be in charge of the analysis of the process.

Defining Indicators

Indicators to be examined in claims audits are different from those used in coding reviews. The detailed work of defining the appropriate indicators is a crucial step that must be completed before any data is retrieved. Analysis of multiple indicators allows a facility to prioritize areas for further examination. To begin with, each organization should establish simple descriptive indicators such as the most frequently billed (top 10, top 50, and so on) APCs and DRGs, average length of stay for each DRG, or number of short-stay admissions. These indicators may be further stratified, or broken out into smaller groups by payer or unit, depending on the needs of the individual facility.

CMI as assigned by HCFA can be used as a crude indicator. CMI for APC is possible but requires attention to appropriate grouping because of wide disparity in APC relative weights and associated resource use and costs.

CMI for inpatient analysis is an indicator of a facility's overall resource use and is driven by ICD-9-CM coding. If complications and comorbidities are either not being coded as they should, or are being coded without supporting documentation, this will result in either an artificially low or high CMI. Comparison of a facility's CMI with those of other similar facilities, or comparison of the CMI in the previous year with the CMI in the current year, may indicate a need to examine the facility's coding accuracy in more depth. There are other factors that affect case mix, but all significant increases or decreases should be closely examined and the reason confirmed. APC case mix is driven by HCPCS/CPT coding and is not affected currently by the selection of the diagnosis code.

Denial or rejection rates also serve as an indicator of how the claims processing system and front-end edits in a facility are working.

Using Comparative Data and Designing Claims Audit Reports

Comparative data is used to assist in the evaluation of indicator results and serve as a guide in determining whether an area should be examined in greater depth.

For example, if 42 percent of an organization's total pneumonia cases are reported as complex pneumonia (DRG 079), and 75 percent of the hospitals in the state, or the nation, bill no more than 30 percent of their pneumonia cases as complex pneumonia, then the organization would be wise to examine the coding of their pneumonia records. In some cases, this may be traced to misinterpretation of coding guidelines or misguided advice provided by a reimbursement optimization consultant about what constitutes bacterial pneumonia.

Comparative data from a state or group of similar facilities will help determine whether an indicator merits further examination. Additional sources of comparative data may include the local PRO, the state hospital association or data commission, state medical societies, or consulting firms.

Many hospitals produce comparative data through the use of HCFA's Medicare Provider Analysis and Review (MEDPAR) file. The MEDPAR file contains data for 100 percent of Medicare beneficiaries using hospital inpatient services. A file of services in one year for a state is available from HCFA for a little more than $1,000.

Ordering information for this file is available from HCFA's Web site at www.hcfa.gov/ stats/pufiles.htm in the Public Use Files catalog. Also available from HCFA's Web site are two files that may be downloaded at no cost. Summary statistics of several years of MEDPAR data are available at www.hcfa.gov/stats/medpar/medpar.htm. The most recent year's CMI values for all hospitals in the nation are available at www.hcfa.gov/stats/pufiles.htm under Payment Rates-Institutional Providers.

Meaningful reports should be developed for displaying and analyzing results of the claims review. After design is completed, specifications for indicators are submitted to the individual or department to be responsible for the extraction of the data from the database used for the claims review. These individuals are often in the information services department or the billing or accounting department.

Compiling the Results

Information systems programs can be written for extraction of the data from appropriate databases. You should consider a time period of at least six months (preferably a year) for an initial claims audit. Extraction of claims information from archived claims may be difficult. To obtain information from claims processed in the preceding 12 to 15 months, you may need to restore data from backup tapes or other media. This requires advance planning and collaboration with the information systems department well in advance of the review.

Most hospitals use indicators that measure performance in areas of investigation by federal agencies. This type of indicator is usually a proportion in which the numerator represents a potentially problematic area, such as a commonly miscoded DRG or a short-stay admission. The denominator represents an appropriate larger group of admissions from which the numerator is drawn. The proportion is then multiplied by 100 to obtain the percentage.

An example of an indicator used to examine an area frequently under federal investigation is the DRG pair. The first DRG in the pair is a higher-weighted DRG susceptible to upcoding. The second DRG in the pair is the DRG that more commonly should have been coded instead of the first DRG. This may occur if coding staff inappropriately designates complications and comorbidities not fully supported by clinical documentation or without concurrence with the physician's diagnostic statement. It can also occur if the physician is "coached" or led by an inappropriate query process to add information to the record that indicates these conditions, although the resource use by the hospital did not increase.

This type of indicator would be calculated to produce the proportion of the first DRG to the sum of the first and second DRG.

A one-day stay for a medical DRG may be suspect for medical necessity and admission appropriateness, but a consistent problem may exist if the proportion of one-day stays is very high in a particular DRG or group of related DRGs. Other ideas for indicators can be found in the Medicare Fiscal Intermediary newsletters, the OIG's Workplans, OIG fraud alerts, and materials from your local PRO.

Once the preliminary list of indicators is agreed upon by the organization stakeholders, the specifications for each indicator are delineated. Specifications are instructions regarding what data elements are required to define the numerator and denominator and where to locate each data element in the information system or database.

Specifications should be thoroughly documented and understood for several reasons. This allows an outside auditing firm to understand how a facility obtained results so they can be compared to the external reviewer's results. This also allows the audit team to consistently replicate the indicators when the time comes for the next auditing period, and it also allows new staff to consistently replicate the indicators.

Interpreting the Results of a Claims Audit

After data collection, analysis must take place to interpret the findings and produce meaningful results. One important fact to remember is that indicators with smaller denominators (less than 30) will yield results that are less stable, meaning they are more subject to random fluctuation. A high percentage in one year could be followed by a very low percentage in the following year. Indicators with denominators greater than or equal to 30 are more stable from year to year, and they represent a facility's more commonly rendered services.

By using the data from the model report, it is possible to make some interpretations of the indicator results for this facility. The comparison data provided represents the median, 10th percentile, and 90th percentile values of the indicator percentages from one large state's group of hospitals for 1999. The median value is the value in the middle of the range of values. The 10th and 90th percentile values define the range in which 80 percent of the group's values fall. Values higher or lower than these percentiles should automatically identify an indicator for further examination.

All four indicators from the example facility are worthwhile for further examination because the denominators are larger than 30. All three DRG-related indicators for the example facility exceed the comparison group's median value, but they are still within the range of values representing 80 percent of facilities in the comparison group. Of the three DRG-related indicators, this facility's proportion of DRG 087 (15 percent) is highest relative to the median of the comparison group (6.3 percent). Further investigation is recommended, which may take the form of a coding audit of a sample or all of the 44 claims billed to DRG 087. The one-day stay indicator result is below the median of the comparison group; however, a problem may exist within a single DRG or group of DRGs, and the data should be stratified according to DRG. There may be a high proportion of one-day stays for DRG 127 (congestive heart failure), for example.

Trend Analysis

Initial audits, whether they are focused on coding practices or claims, will provide a baseline or starting point value that can be used to compare to all subsequent measurements. To compare subsequent measurements to the baseline, you should develop a process to allow collection and analysis of measurements made over time. Collecting the measurements made over time in a spreadsheet and plotting them on a line graph is one technique that may be used. Statistical process control charts represent another tool for this task. Control charts to be monitored on a regular basis can be constructed for each indicator, and the calculation of upper and lower control limits will signal when a process is "out of control."

Using Audit Tools for Coding or Claims Review

Use of an audit tool provides consistency in data collection and facilitates collection of required data.

Audit tools for coding review can be used to evaluate simple coding errors and complex errors that affect the DRG assignment. They can be used to identify problems in coding, DRG, or APC assignments or to monitor improvement in such assignments identified previously. Although the instructions are written as if you are performing a postpayment review, you could also adapt the form to a prepayment review.

Preparation for Use of Audit Tools

When review of a group of similar cases (like diagnoses and procedures) is planned, auditors are recommended to review related coding conventions and guidelines specific to that clinical area. It is helpful to be aware of any coding problems that can occur by reviewing the OIG fraud alerts or looking at past areas of concern.

Recording Record, Claim Review, and Findings Using the Audit Tools

Auditors compare the medical record to the claim to ensure that the documentation matches what was reported on the claim form.

If the medical record does not match the claim in terms of the patient name, admission date, physician orders, or provider number, further action is necessary. Consultation with the physician may be needed, and a request to provide an addendum to the medical record, correct the claim, and rebill the services, or take other action, may also be required. Documentation after discharge for the express purpose of seeking reimbursement and not contributing to patient care may be a questionable practice.

The auditor should review the medical record to ensure that the diagnosis reported as the principal diagnosis meets UHDDS definitions. It must have been present at admission, been a principal reason for admission, and received treatment or evaluation during the stay. If several diagnoses meet all of these requirements, and sequencing guidelines do not require you to code one over the others, you may select any one of the diagnoses as the principal diagnosis. If the principal diagnosis was chosen incorrectly, the correct diagnosis should be determined. If this can be determined by using official coding conventions and guidelines, you do not necessarily have to obtain physician consultation, as long the record clearly supports this action. If the documentation in the medical record is unclear, consultation with the attending physician is mandatory to obtain answers to questions about the appropriateness of the codes reported. Best practices suggest that physicians be notified any time the code reporting is at variance with the final diagnostic statement at discharge. If any changes affect the DRG, resubmission of the claim is required. The hospital must ensure that physician clarification is documented in the medical record in an addendum. If a pattern of rebilling is noted for specific physicians or for specific types of cases, an indicator should be established and a corrective action plan implemented.

In addition to diagnosis and procedure verification with the medical record to determine if the patient's age and discharge status were billed correctly, incorrect designation of discharge status or age can result in incorrect DRG assignment. Problems in this area should also be trended and corrective action taken. Discharge status errors sometimes occur owing to a mapping error between the abstracting system and the claims generation process.

For outpatient records, the reason for the visit should be reported and corresponding diagnoses indicated to support justification of the medical necessity for each service rendered. Modifiers should be applied appropriately when indicated, and all CPT and Level II HCPCS codes assigned should be verified, whether they are selected by coding staff or posted by the chargemaster.

When coding affects the DRG or APC payments, auditors should classify the cause of changes by using the problem areas provided on the audit form. Also, note the original and revised DRG or APCs and the difference in reimbursement. This will allow you to track whether your coding errors involving claims are resulting in over- or underpayments.

Follow-up of Audit Tool Completion

Individual audit results are maintained to identify any undesirable patterns and trends. Once a problem or opportunity for improvement has been identified, an organization is expected to implement corrective action to protect its corporate integrity. After improvement has been noted, it is important to focus on new areas, being sure to periodically check old problems to ensure that improvement is sustained.

Credibility demands that the person completing the audit form sign and date it. This demonstrates that qualified staff is performing audits to ensure an effective compliance program committed to following regulatory requirements and payment rules. It also allows accountability tracking and facilitates quality review of the audit process. Also, should a government investigation occur in the future, this documentation would demonstrate that auditing predated the investigation, and there was a process in place to identify problems and take corrective action. Consultation with legal counsel is recommended regarding how to structure and document this type of information.

Results and Recommendations

Audits must result in corrective action specific to the problems identified in the reviews. Any problem involving significant overpayment, confirmed upcoding, questionable medical necessity trends, or any issues with potential for inaccurate payment must be referred to the compliance office or compliance committee for follow-up. On the basis of audit outcomes, corrective action may include designing a form to be used by physicians for documenting final diagnoses, providing physician education on medical record documentation and coding, updating coding books, providing feedback to the coding staff involved, implementing prebilling coding validation, or other steps specific to the problem.

Conclusion

Following the suggestions and guidelines set forth in this paper will produce an effective compliance audit process for coding and reimbursement and the related documentation supporting those activities.

Resource List

"2001 OIG Workplan" is available at www.dhhs.gov/progorg/wrkpln/2001/hcfa.pdf.

"Improper Fiscal Year 2000 Medicare Fee-for-Service Payments" is available at www.dhhs.gov/progorg/oas/reports/afma/a0002000.pdf.

Osborne, Carole E. "DRG Analysis Reveals Potential Problems, Trends." *Journal of the American Health Information Management Association* 72, no. 7 (2001): 78–83.

"Payment Error Prevention Program," Arkansas Foundation for Medical Care, 2001. (Many states have similar reference materials available from the PRO under contract by the Medicare Intermediary.)

"Practice Brief." *Journal of the American Health Information Management Association* 72, no. 7 (2001): 64A–64C.

Prophet, Sue. *Health Information Management Compliance: A Model Program for Healthcare Organizations.* Chicago: AHIMA, 2000.

Russo, Ruthann. Fernald, Frances (Managing Editor). *A Guide to Auditing Health Care Billing Practices.* Washington, DC: Atlantic Information Services, Inc., 2001.

Endnotes

1. The OIG Workplan is available at http://www.dhhs.gov/progorg/wrkpln/2001/hcfa.pdf.

2. Russo, Ruthann. Fernald, Frances (Managing Editor). *A Guide to Auditing Health Care Billing Practices.* Washington, DC: Atlantic Information Services, Inc., 2001.

3. www.dhhs.gov/progorg

4. Osborne, Carole E. "DRG Analysis Reveals Potential Problems, Trends." *Journal of the American Health Information Management Association* 72, no. 7 (2001): 78–83.

Appendix G

Sample Audit Worksheets, Forms, and Tools

Sample audit forms are from *Health Information Management Compliance: A Model Program for Healthcare Organizations*. Chicago: AHIMA, 2000.

Compliance Coding Review
Daily Worksheet

INPATIENT CASES

Date of Review: _____

Name	Med Rec #	D/C Date	Coder	Date Coded	Original DRG	Revised DRG	Positive Impact	Negative Impact	Comment	Variation Type

Source: Bowman, Sue. 2008. *Health Information Management Compliance: Guidelines for Preventing Fraud and Abuse, 4th ed.* Chicago: AHIMA.

Inpatient Review
Variations by Coder

Date of Review: _____

VARIATION TYPE

Inaccurate sequencing or specificity prin dx, affect   _____
DRG

Inaccurate sequencing or specificity prin dx, no affect   _____
DRG

Omission CC, affect DRG   _____

Omission CC, no affect DRG   _____

Inaccurate prin procedure, affect DRG   _____

Omission procedure, affect DRG   _____

More specific coding of dx or proc, no affect DRG   _____

Inaccurate coding   _____

Compliance Audit

MR # : _____

Date of Surgery: _____

Procedure: _____

Diagnosis: _____

Reviewer agrees with codes assigned to record?

❏ Yes   ❏ No

Revised ICD-9-CM Diagnosis Codes:

_____

_____

Revised CPT Procedure Code/ICD-9-CM Procedure Code:

_____

_____

Record Completeness: (Medical necessity for procedure/treatment documented?)

❏ All complete   ❏ Areas not completed or deficient (document below)

BILLING REVIEW:

| | ❏ Yes | ❏ No |

Registration information complete and form signed by patient/other?

Deficiencies:

_____

| | ❏ Yes | ❏ No |

If Medicare, CCI edits applied to case where applicable?

Deficiencies:

_____

If resubmitted to carrier based on code/CCI edit changes, was payment appropriately refunded or additional billed?

_____

Submit case to Compliance Committee for further review and discussion?   ❏ Yes   ❏ No

_____   _____
Reviewer   Date

Coding Audit Summary

Date: _____   Reviewed by: _____

Review Type: MR #
_____   _____

Name: Account #
_____   _____

FC: Admit/DC Date:
_____   _____

LOS: Disposition:
_____   _____

Attending Phys: Surgeon/Consult:
_____   _____

Original Dx Codes:	Revised Dx Codes:	Type of Change:
1. _____	1. _____	Pr Dx
2. _____	2. _____	
		/_____/
3. _____	3. _____	
4. _____	4. _____	CC Dx
5. _____	5. _____	/_____/
6. _____	6. _____	2nd Dx
7. _____	7. _____	/_____/
8. _____	8. _____	Add Dx
9. _____	9. _____	/_____/
		Del Dx
		/_____/
		Other
		/_____/

Original Procedure Codes:	Revised Procedure Codes:	Type of Change:
1. _____	1. _____	
2. _____	2. _____	Pr Proc
3. _____	3. _____	/_____/
4. _____	4. _____	Sig Proc
5. _____	5. _____	/_____/
6. _____	6. _____	2nd Proc
7. _____	7. _____	/_____/
8. _____	8. _____	Add Proc
9. _____	9. _____	/_____/
		Del Proc
		/_____/
		Other
		/_____/

Date Coded: Date of D/S: Coder:

_____   _____   _____

Documentation Issues: **Physician(s):**

_____

_____

_____

_____

Findings/Recommendations:

_____

_____

_____

_____

_____

DRG Change: Yes_____   No _____

Original DRG: Weight: Reimbursement:

_____   _____   _____

Revised DRG: Weight: Reimbursement:

_____   _____   _____

Rebilling Date: Wt. Diff: Adjustment:

_____   _____   _____

Coding Audit Review Sheet

Coder:_____

Type of Review (IP,OP,ER):_____

Date of Review: _____

Medical Record # :_____

Discharge Date: _____

Initial Coding	Reviewer's Recommendations

Principal Diagnosis
   A. Chosen and coded correctly   _____

   B. Chosen correctly, coded incorrectly   _____

   C. Chosen incorrectly, coded correctly   _____

   D. Chosen and coded incorrectly   _____

Secondary Diagnoses
   A. Chosen and coded correctly   _____

   B. Chosen correctly, coded incorrectly   _____

   C. Chosen incorrectly, coded correctly   _____

   D. Chosen and coded incorrectly   _____

Principal Procedure
   A. Chosen and coded correctly   _____

   B. Chosen correctly, coded incorrectly   _____

   C. Chosen incorrectly, coded correctly   _____

   D. Chosen and coded incorrectly   _____

Secondary Procedures
   A. Chosen and coded correctly   _____

   B. Chosen correctly, coded incorrectly   _____

   C. Chosen incorrectly, coded correctly   _____

   D. Chosen and coded incorrectly   _____

DRG
   A. Chosen and coded correctly   _____

   B. Chosen correctly, coded incorrectly   _____

   C. Chosen incorrectly, coded correctly   _____

   D. Chosen and coded incorrectly   _____

Audit Summary

Total number of records in sample:

	#	%
Principal Diagnosis (total)		
A. Chosen and coded correctly	_____	_____
B. Chosen correctly, coded incorrectly	_____	_____
C. Chosen incorrectly and coded correctly	_____	_____
D. Chosen and coded incorrectly	_____	_____
Secondary diagnoses found/total possible secondary diagnoses (total)		
A. All found	_____	_____
B. All not found: # missed	_____	_____
Secondary diagnoses coded/total possible secondary diagnoses (total)		
A. All coded correctly	_____	_____
B. All codes not correct: # missed	_____	_____
Principal Procedure (total)		
A. Chosen and coded correctly	_____	_____
B. Chosen correctly, coded incorrectly	_____	_____
C. Chosen incorrectly and coded correctly	_____	_____
D. Chosen and coded incorrectly	_____	_____

Secondary procedures found/total possible secondary procedures (total)

    A. All found   _____   _____

    B. All not found: # missed   _____   _____

Secondary procedures coded/total possible secondary procedures (total)

    A. All coded correctly   _____   _____

    B. All codes not correct: # missed _____   _____

DRG (total)

    A. DRGs all correct   _____

    B. DRGs not correct   _____

        1. Due to principal diagnosis   _____

        2. Due to secondary diagnosis _____

        3. Due to principal procedure   _____

        4. Due to secondary procedure _____

CPT (total)

    A. All CPT codes correct   _____

    B. All CPT codes not correct: # wrong _____

Total records coded completely correctly   _____

Total possible choices   _____

Total actual correct   _____

Coding Compliance Review – Inpatient Summary

Name: _____   Age: _____   ADM: _____

MR # : _____   Sex: _____   DISCH: _____

ACCT # : _____   MD: _____   Facility: _____

HIC # : _____   LOS: _____   Payer: _____

Original Description and
Codes
Diagnosis   DRG
_____

Revised Description and
Codes
Diagnosis   DRG
_____

Original	Revised	Variance Type:		
1.	1.	*Variance Type:*		
		PrDx		Chg
2.	2.	/___/		
		ReSeq		PrDx
3.	3.	/___/		
		Add	2nd	Dx
4.	4.	/___/		
		Chg	2nd	Dx
5.	5.	/___/		
		PrProc		Chg
6.	6.	/___/		
		Chg	2nd	Proc
7.	7.	/___/		
		Add		Proc
8.	8.	/___/		
		Other		
9.	9.	/___/		
10.	10.			

Operative Description and Codes

1. _____

2. _____

3. _____

4. _____

5. _____

6. _____

Operative Description and Codes

1. _____

2. _____

3. _____

4. _____

5. _____

6. _____

Disposition Code: _____

Disposition Code: _____

Summary Findings:

_____

_____

_____

Recommendations:

_____

_____

_____

_____

Date Reviewed: _____

Reviewer: _____

Orig. DRG Wt.: _____

Pmt: _____

Date sent to Rebill HIM for: _____

Revised DRG Wt.: _____

Pmt.: _____

Diff.: _____

Dictation:
　DxSum (dict): _____

　Typed _____

H+P (dict): _____

Typed _____

Oper. (dict): _____

Typed _____

Audit Tool Elements excerpted from PRO PEPP Manual (Arkansas Foundation for Medical Care)

Yes/No

Does the medical record:

- Match the claim being reviewed?
- Contain an inpatient order for the date of admission and the level of care billed?
- Match the provider number billed (e.g., PPS vs. Non-PPS)?

Is the principal diagnosis:

- Present on admission?
- A principal reason for admission?
- Treated or evaluated during the stay?

Is documentation present to support secondary diagnoses and complications/comorbidities billed?

Are there any that are present, but not reported, that affect DRG assignment?

Is documentation present to support procedures billed? Procedures omitted that would affect the DRG?

Patient's age and discharge status accurate?

Are there other coding errors?

- Code does not match actual dx or procedure.
- Code lacks specificity.
- Sequencing is incorrect.
- Coding does not follow ICD-9-CM coding conventions.
- Coding does not follow *Coding Clinic* guidelines.

What is the cause of any DRG change?

(List examples from above to check off.)

Abbreviations

AFDC: *Aid to Families with Dependent Children.* One of the CMS Medicaid eligibility categories.

AHA: *American Hospital Association.* A national association that supports member institutions. For health information, the AHA is the clearinghouse for ICD-9-CM coding issues. AHA is one of the four Cooperating Parties on policy development for the use of ICD-9-CM.

AHIMA: *American Health Information Management Association.* A professional organization for HIM professionals. AHIMA provides seminars and publications supporting the use of ICD-9-CM. It is one of the four Cooperating Parties that approve official coding policy.

AHRQ: *Agency for Healthcare Research and Quality.* The branch of the United States Public Health Service that supports general health research and distributes research findings and treatment guidelines with the goal of improving the quality, appropriateness, and effectiveness of healthcare services.

AMA: *American Medical Association.* An association for physicians that promotes the science and art of medicine. The AMA maintains and publishes the *Current Procedural Terminology* (CPT) coding system.

AP-DRGs: *All-patient diagnosis-related groups.* A case-mix system developed by 3M and used in a number of state reimbursement systems to classify non-Medicare discharges for reimbursement purposes.

APR-DRGs: *All-patient refined diagnosis-related groups.* A case mix system developed by 3M that includes four distinct subclasses (minor, moderate, major, and extreme) based on the severity of the patient's illness.

BBA: *Balanced Budget Act of 1997.* Public Law 105-33 enacted by Congress on August 5, 1997, that mandated a number of additions, deletions, and revisions to the original Medicare and Medicaid legislation; the legislation that added penalties for healthcare fraud and abuse to the Medicare and Medicaid programs.

BBRA: *Balanced Budget Refinement Act of 1999.* The amended version of the Balanced Budget Act of 1997 that authorizes implementation of a per-discharge prospective payment system for care provided to Medicare beneficiaries by inpatient rehabilitation facilities.

CC: *Complication/comorbidity.* A *complication* is a condition arising after the beginning of hospital observation and treatment that modifies the course of the patient's illness or the medical care required. A *comorbidity* is a preexisting condition that will, because of its presence with a specific principal diagnosis, cause an increase in the patient's length of stay by at least one day in 75 percent of cases. Complications and comorbidities generally require coding as additional diagnoses and may affect DRG assignment.

CDS: *Clinical documentation specialists.* Coding professionals and nurses who work on the patient floors or alongside the physicians in the clinic setting.

CHAMPUS: *Civilian Health and Medical Program—Uniformed Services.* A federal program providing supplementary civilian-sector hospital and medical services beyond that which is available in military treatment facilities to military dependents, retirees and their dependents, and certain others. Now known as TRICARE.

CHAMPVA: *Civilian Health and Medical Program—Veterans Administration.* The federal healthcare benefits program for dependents of veterans rated by the Veterans Administration as having a total and permanent disability, for survivors of veterans who died from VA-rated service-connected conditions or who were rated permanently and totally disabled at the time of death from a VA-rated service-connected condition, and for survivors of persons who died in the line of duty.

CMI: *Case-mix index.* The average relative weight of all cases treated at a given facility or by a given physician, which reflects the resource intensity or clinical severity of a specific group in relation to the other groups in the classification system; calculated by dividing the sum of the weights of diagnosis-related groups for patients discharged during a given period divided by the total number of patients discharged.

CMS: *Centers for Medicare and Medicaid Services.* Formerly known as HCFA, this government agency is responsible for administration of the Medicare and Medicaid programs. CMS is one of the four Cooperating Parties that approve official coding policy.

COBRA: *Consolidated Omnibus Budget Reconciliation Act of 1975.* The federal law requiring every hospital that participates in Medicare and has an emergency department to treat any patient in an emergency condition or active labor, whether or not the patient is covered by Medicare and regardless of the patient's ability to pay; COBRA also requires employers to provide continuation benefits to specified workers and families who have been terminated but previously had healthcare insurance benefits.

CPG: *Compliance program guidance.* The information provided by the OIG to help healthcare organizations develop internal controls that promote adherence to applicable federal and state guidelines.

DRA: *Deficit Reduction Act of 2005.* Legislation that provides states the flexibility to reform their Medicaid programs.

DRG: *Diagnosis-related group.* DRGs represent a classification system that categorizes patients who are medically related with respect to their diagnoses and treatments and are statistically similar in their lengths of stay. See MS-DRG.

DME: *Durable medical equipment.* Medical equipment designed for long-term use in the home, including eyeglasses, hearing aids, surgical appliances and supplies, orthotics and prostheses, and bulk and cylinder oxygen.

DMERC: *Durable medical equipment regional carrier.* A fiscal intermediary designated to process claims for durable medical equipment.

FI: *Fiscal intermediary.* An organization that contracts with the Centers for Medicare and Medicaid Services to serve as the financial agent between providers and the federal government in the local administration of Medicare Part A claims.

FPL: *Federal poverty level.* The income qualification threshold established by the federal government for certain government entitlement programs.

HHS: *Department of Health and Human Services.* A government executive branch department that oversees CMS's administration of the Medicare and Medicaid programs and the work of many other government agencies related to healthcare.

HIMS: *Health information management services.* One of several names for the health record department. This name is meant to provide a better description of the function of the department, which is the management of health information.

HIPAA: *Health Insurance Portability and Accountability Act of 1996.* The federal legislation enacted to provide continuity of health coverage, control fraud and abuse in healthcare, reduce healthcare costs, and guarantee the security and privacy of health information. The act limits exclusion for preexisting medical conditions, prohibits discrimination against employees and dependents based on health status, guarantees availability of health insurance to small employers, and guarantees renewability of insurance to all employees regardless of size.

HMO: *Health maintenance organization.* Entity that combines the provision of healthcare insurance and the delivery of healthcare services, characterized by: (1) organized healthcare delivery system to a geographic area, (2) set of basic and supplemental health maintenance and treatment services, (3) voluntarily enrolled members, and (4) predetermined fixed, periodic prepayments for members' coverage.

HPMP: *Hospital Payment Monitoring Program.* A program designed to measure, monitor, and reduce the incidence of improper fee-for-service inpatient payments. Replaced the Payment Error Prevention Program (PEPP).

ICD-9-CM: *International Classification of Diseases, 9th Revision, Clinical Modification for Use in the United States.* A diagnostic and procedural classification system published by NCHS and CMS in cooperation with the World Health Organization.

ICD-10: *International Classification of Diseases, 10th Revision.* The most recent update of the ICD diagnostic and procedural classification system, currently in use in some parts of the world. Clinical modification (ICD-10-CM) is being developed for implementation in the United States.

ICD-10-PCS: *International Classification of Diseases, 10th Revision, Procedural Classification System.* Procedural classification system being developed in conjunction with ICD-10.

IPA: *Individual practice association, independent physician association, independent practice association, or independent provider association.* A form of HMO that consists of a group of physicians who form together as a legal corporation to provide care for the HMO patients.

IPF: *Inpatient psychiatric facility.* An inpatient facility or unit of an existing hospital that specializes in inpatient treatment for psychiatric disorders.

IRF: *Inpatient rehabilitation facility.* An inpatient facility or unit that specializes in post–acute care services for rehabilitation purposes.

IRVEN: *Inpatient Rehabilitation Validation and Entry.* A computerized data-entry system used by inpatient rehabilitation facilities.

LCD: *Local coverage determination.* Coverage rules, at a fiscal intermediary (FI) or carrier level, that provide information on what diagnoses justify the medical necessity of a test.

LMRPs: *Local medical review policies.* Documents that define Medicare coverage of outpatient services via lists of diagnoses defined as medically reasonable and necessary for the services provided.

LOS: *Length of stay.* The total number of patient days for an inpatient episode, calculated by subtracting the date of admission from the date of discharge.

MA: *Medicare Advantage (Medicare Part C).* A PPO-type of coverage for Medicare beneficiaries that offers options such as regional PPOs and specialized health plans for certain diagnoses.

MAC: *Medicare Administrative Contractor.* The Medicare Prescription Drug, Improvement and Modernization Act of 2003 (MMA) allowed CMS to make significant changes to Medicare's administrative structure. CMS is integrating administration of Medicare Parts A (Fiscal Intermediaries/FI) and B (Carriers) for the fee-for-service benefit into Medicare Administrative Contractors (MACs).

MA-PD: *Medicare Advantage-Prescription Drug.* The Medicare plan that includes medication coverage.

MCC: *Major Complication/Comorbidity* A *complication* is a condition arising after the beginning of hospital observation and treatment that modifies the course of the patient's illness or the medical care required. A *comorbidity* is a preexisting condition that will, because of its presence with a specific principal diagnosis, cause an increase in the patient's length of stay by at least one day in 75 percent of cases. Medicare has designated certain conditions as *MCCs (major complications/comorbidities)* that when present as a secondary diagnosis have a greater impact on length of stay and/or resources used to care for the patient and may affect MS-DRG Assignment.

MDC: *Major diagnostic category.* A part of the DRG system that divides all possible principal diagnoses into twenty-five mutually exclusive areas. MDCs were formed to ensure that MS-DRGs would be clinically coherent.

MDHs: *Medicare-dependent rural hospitals.* Facilities that are paid based on a formula of DRG rate or on their costs for specific time periods, whichever is higher.

MMA: *Medicare Prescription Drug, Improvement, and Modernization Act (MMA) of 2003.* Major changes to the Medicare program, including creation of Medicare Part D drug benefit (2006), creation of Health Savings Accounts (HSAs) and increased payments to Medicare HMOs.

MS-DRG: *Medicare Severity Adjusted Diagnosis Related Group.* MS-DRGs were the significant update by Medicare in 2008 to better account for patients' severity of illness. They represent a classification system that categorizes patients who are medically related with respect to their diagnoses and treatments and are statistically similar in their lengths of stay.

MSP: *Medicare secondary payer.* One of the edits in the outpatient and inpatient code editors that reviews claims to determine if the claim should be paid by another form of insurance, such as workers' compensation or private insurance in the event of a traffic accident.

NCQA: *National Committee for Quality Assurance.* A private not-for-profit accreditation organization whose mission is to evaluate and report on the quality of managed care organizations in the United States.

NCD: *National coverage determination.* The equivalent of an LCD at the national level.

NCHS: *National Center for Health Statistics.* A government agency that works with CMS to revise ICD-9-CM codes and approve official coding policy. NCHS is one of the four Cooperating Parties that approve official coding policy.

NCVHS: *National Committee on Vital and Health Statistics.* A public policy advisory board that recommends policy to the National Center for Health Statistics and other health-related federal programs.

OBRA: *Omnibus Budget Reconciliation Act of 1986.* A federal law that requires outpatient visits, either medical or surgical, to be reported using ICD-9-CM and HCPCS for outpatient services billing.

OIG: *Office of the Inspector General.* The office through which the federal government established compliance plans for the healthcare industry.

P4P: *Pay for performance.* A movement toward reimbursing physicians proportionate to the quality of care. Electronic health records (EHRs) can improve quality of care by having functions such as automatic pop-up reminders during electronic charting. Reminders can be programmed into EHR systems to address such issues as contraindications and drug interactions triggered by the data entered. Another aspect of P4P is related to outcomes documented during subsequent patient visits.

PDP: *Prescription drug plan.* Patients who chose to remain in the traditional Medicare coverage plans will have the option of joining a PDP to obtain drug benefits for an additional charge.

PHO: *Physician–hospital organization.* An IPA where physicians and hospital(s) join together to provide contracted services. In a PHO, both the hospital and the physician practices share in the risk associated with prepayment of services.

PIP-DCG: *Principal inpatient diagnostic cost group.* A model designed to calculate each beneficiary's relative risk in terms of overall Medicare expenditures.

POA: *Present On Admission.* The UB-04 form has an additional field for all diagnoses codes to indicate whether the condition was present on admission. Instructions for accurately reporting conditions as POA are included in the ICD-9-CM Official Coding Guidelines.

PPS: *Prospective payment system.* A government reimbursement plan implemented in 1983 to control the cost of inpatient hospital services to Medicare recipients. Payments were set at a flat rate rather than on a fee-for-service or per day basis.

RIC: *Rehabilitation impairment category.* A group reflective of the primary need for rehabilitation care.

QIO: *Quality improvement organization.* CMS contracts with private medical review organizations to ensure that the government pays only for medically necessary, appropriate, and high-quality healthcare services. QIOs conduct DRG validations to compare the hospital's coding of the case on the claim with the attending physician's documentation in the health record.

SCHs: *Sole community hospitals.* Small facilities that are paid based on a formula of DRG rate or on their costs for specific time periods, whichever is higher.

SCHIP: *State Children's Health Insurance Program.* The children's healthcare program implemented as part of the Balanced Budget Act of 1997; sometimes referred to as the Children's Health Insurance Program, or CHIP.

SOW: *Scope of work.* The QIOs' contract with CMS that specifies the goals and topics for review.

SSI: *Supplemental Security Income.* One of the CMS Medicaid eligibility categories.

TEFRA: *Tax Equity and Fiscal Responsibility Act of 1982.* The federal legislation that modified Medicare's retrospective reimbursement system for inpatient hospital stays by requiring implementation of diagnosis-related groups and the acute care prospective payment system.

UB-04: *Uniform Bill-2004.* Updated in 2004, this single uniform bill consolidated the numerous forms that hospitals were using to submit bills to third-party payers. The HIM department supplies the clinical data that are placed on the form and ensures their accuracy.

UCDS: *Uniform Clinical Data Set.* A standard set of data about each hospitalization. The UCDS was developed to form the foundation for a new review methodology. The goal is to move from retrospective case-by-case review to a system based on computerized analysis of large databases, which will identify patterns of use and outcome.

UHDDS: *Uniform Hospital Discharge Data Set.* A minimum common core of data on individual hospital discharges in the Medicare and Medicaid programs. Its purpose is to provide uniformity and comparability in hospital discharge data.

UR: *Utilization review.* The process of determining whether the medical care provided to a specific patient is necessary according to preestablished objective screening criteria at time frames specified in the organization's utilization management plan.

VBP: *Value-based purchasing.* Links payment more directly to the quality of care provided. CMS has launched VBP initiatives in hospitals, physician offices, nursing homes, home health services, and dialysis facilities.

Annotated Bibliography

American Health Information Management Association. 1990 to present. Coding notes and clinical notes, *Journal of American Health Information Management Association.* A monthly column in the *Journal of AHIMA* that features coding advice, the latest peer review organization information, and clinical disease discussions.

American Hospital Association. 1984 to present. *Coding Clinic for ICD-9-CM.* **Chicago: AHA.** Published quarterly by the AHA, *Coding Clinic* responds to questions from coders across the country and contains official coding policy, including the official guidelines for ICD-9-CM coding practices. Its content is cleared by the Cooperating Parties prior to publication.

Beers, Mark H. 2006. *Merck Manual, 18th edition.* **Robert S. Porter and Thomas V. Jones, editors. Whitehouse Station, NJ: Merck.** A compendium by body system of common diseases and health problems. Each disease is presented with typical signs, laboratory tests usually performed to affirm the diagnosis, and potential treatment options.

Bowman, Sue. 2008. *Health Information Management Compliance: Guidelines for Preventing Fraud and Abuse, 4th ed.* **Chicago: AHIMA.** This resource for effective compliance programs in all healthcare settings delivers the latest compliance research and trends in an easy-to-understand format. It includes sample auditing and monitoring tools, guidelines for documentation within existing systems, and structures for designing a compliance program, and information on how to prepare for an audit.

Code Write. **Chicago: AHIMA.** The monthly newsletter of the Coding Community of Practice (CoP). Available on the Coding CoP at www.ahima.org/. *Code Write* features articles about issues relevant to the community of professional clinical coders.

Dorland. 2007. *Dorland's Illustrated Medical Dictionary, 31st edition.* **Philadelphia: W.B. Saunders.** A traditional medical dictionary used by most transcriptionists. It contains anatomic and disease-oriented illustrations. The book is usually updated annually. Purchase of the new edition of this book every other year or every two years is generally acceptable.

Fischbach, Frances. 2003. *A Manual of Laboratory Diagnostic Tests, 7th edition.* **Philadelphia: Lippincott Williams & Wilkins.** A laboratory manual that presents lab tests, normal ranges, abnormal ranges, and what the abnormal value indicates. Any manual providing this information would be adequate.

Gahart, Betty L., and Adrienne Nazareno. 2004. *2005 Intravenous Medications: A Handbook for Nurses and Allied Health Professionals, 21st edition.* St. Louis: Mosby. A reference and review guide to indications, potential side effects, dosages, and implications for use of drugs administered intravenously.

McPhee, Stephen J., Papadakis, Maxine A., and Lawrence M. Tierney. 2006. *Current Medical Diagnosis and Treatment 2007, 46th edition.* New York: McGraw-Hill Professional Publishing. An annual publication that presents most medical illnesses by body system with a straightforward discussion outlining symptoms, differential diagnoses, and typical treatment protocols. Purchasing this text every other year or every two years is generally adequate.

Schraffenberger, Lou Ann. 2007. *Basic ICD-9-CM Coding.* Chicago: AHIMA. This annual publication offers basic coding instruction, including *Coding Clinic* guidelines. The most current edition should be kept available to coders.

Scott, Karen S. 2008. *Medical Coding for Non-coders: Understanding Coding and Reimbursement in Today's Healthcare Industry.* Chicago: AHIMA. This book delivers an introduction to medical coding for non-coding healthcare professionals. An overview of coding and reimbursement systems provides a full understanding of code sets, billing, and fraudulent coding.

Springhouse. 2007. *Springhouse Nurse's Drug Guide 2008.* Ambler, PA: Lippincott Williams & Wilkins. A reference guide to medication, similar to *Physicians' Desk Reference.*

Thomson Healthcare. 2008. *Physicians' Desk Reference, 62nd edition.* Montvale, NJ: Thompson Healthcare. The traditional reference manual for pharmacies. It identifies most drugs, their indications, contraindications, dosages, and such. Any current manual that supplies similar information is required.

3M/Health Information Systems. 2003. *Diagnosis Related Groups Definitions Manual.* Current Version. Salt Lake City: 3M/Health Information Systems. The official documentation for the Medicare grouper in use for the current fiscal year of the prospective payment system.

U.S. Government. 2004. *International Classification of Diseases, Clinical Modification for Use in the United States.* Washington, DC: U.S. Government Printing Office. Everyone who codes manually should have an updated codebook. If an encoder is used, at least one manual should be available for reference. Changes are effective every October 1.

Way, Lawrence, and Gerard M. Doherty. 2002. *Current Surgical Diagnosis and Treatment, 11th edition.* Norwalk, CT: Appleton and Lange. An annual publication that presents most surgical illnesses by body system with a straightforward discussion outlining symptoms, surgical options, and typical complications. Purchasing this text every other year or every two years is generally adequate.

Wilson, Donna D. 2008. Benchmarking to Improve Coding Accuracy and Productivity. Rose Dunn, editor. Chicago: AHIMA. In recognition of the need to benchmark coding processes, FORE/AHIMA conducted a Coding Benchmark Survey that assessed current coding practices in use by AHIMA members in a variety of organizations—with and without EHRs—across the United States to establish a baseline for coding practices. This book outlines the results of the survey and provides recommendations for best practices in coding quality and productivity.

References

AHIMA Coding Products and Services Team. 2003 (July/August). Practice brief: Managing and improving data quality. *Journal of American Health Information Management Association* 74(7):64A–C.

AHIMA. 2008a. Coding resources. Available online from http://www.ahima.org/coding/coding_resources.asp.

AHIMA. 2008b. Certifications. Available online from http://www.ahima.org/certification/.

American Hospital Association. 1991–2007. *Coding Clinic for ICD-9-CM.* Chicago: AHA.

American Society of Plastic Surgeons. 2008. Available online from http://www.plasticsurgery.org.

Bryant, Gloryanne. 2007 (March). *CodeWrite Community News*, Chicago: AHIMA.

Buff, Elizabeth Logan, and Samuel Hohmann. 1999 (May). Navigating from data to excellence. *Journal of American Health Information Management Association* 70(5): 44–48.

Cassidy, Bonnie, et al. 1998. Practice brief: Data quality management model. *Journal of American Health Information Management Association* 69(6).

Centers for Disease Control. 2008 (Jan. 11). ICD-9-CM coordination and maintenance committee. Available online from http://www.cdc.gov/nchs/about/otheract/icd9/maint/maint.htm.

Centers for Medicare & Medicaid Services. 2008a. Acute inpatient PPS overview: Steps in Determining a PPS Payment. Available online from http://www.cms.hhs.gov/AcuteInpatientPPS/02_stepspps.asp#TopOfPage.

Centers for Medicare & Medicaid Services. 2008b (January). Long-term care hospital prospective payment system. Interrupted stay fact sheet. Available online from http://www.cms.hhs.gov/MLNProducts/downloads/LTCH-IntStay.pdf.

Centers for Medicare & Medicaid Services. 2008c (January). Long-term care hospital prospective payment system. Short stay outliers fact sheet. Available online from http://www.cms.hhs.gov/MLNProducts/downloads/LTCH-ShortStay.pdf.

Centers for Medicare & Medicaid Services. 2007a. Medicare Benefit Policy Manual, Chapter 1—Inpatient Hospital Services Covered Under Part A. Available online from http://www.cms.hhs.gov/manuals/Downloads/bp102c01.pdf.

Centers for Medicare & Medicaid Services. 2007b (May 14). Office of Public Affairs, Press release: Medicare pay for performance (P4P) initiatives. Available online from http://www.cms.hhs.gov/apps/media/press/release.asp?Counter=1343.

Centers for Medicare & Medicaid Services. 2007c (Jan. 17). Hospital pay-for-performance workgroup: Medicare hospital value-based purchasing plan development. Issues paper, 1st public listening session. Available online from http://www.cms.hhs.gov/AcuteInpatientPPS/downloads/hospital_VBP_plan_issues_paper.pdf.

Centers for Medicare & Medicaid Services. 2007d (Aug. 22). Changes to the Hospital Inpatient Prospective Payment Systems and Fiscal Year 2008 Rates; Final Rule. 42 CFR Parts 411, 412, 413, and 489. *Federal Register* 72(162):47130–48175. Available online from http://a257.g.akamaitech.net/7/257/2422/01jan20071800/edocket.access.gpo.gov/2007/pdf/07-3820.pdf.

Centers for Medicare & Medicaid Services. 2007e (May 3). Medicare Program; Proposed Changes to the Hospital Inpatient Prospective Payment Systems and Fiscal Year 2008 Rates. *Federal Register* 72(85):24779–24828.

Centers for Medicare & Medicaid Services. 2007f (Oct. 1). Long term care hospital PPS, FY 2008 MS-LTC-DRG File. Available online from http://www.cms.hhs.gov/LongTermCareHospitalPPS/06_ltcdrg.asp#TopOfPage.

Centers for Medicare & Medicaid Services. 2007g (Aug. 7) Medicare Program; Inpatient Rehabilitation Facility Prospective Payment. System for Federal Fiscal Year 2008; Final Rule. 42 CFR Part 412. *Federal Register* 72(151):44283-44335. Available online from http://www.cms.hhs.gov/quarterlyproviderupdates/downloads/cms1551f.pdf.

Centers for Medicare & Medicaid Services. 2007h (Oct. 2). Inpatient rehabilitation facility PPS software. Available online from http://www.cms.hhs.gov/InpatientRehabFacPPS/06_Software.asp#TopOfPage.

Centers for Medicare & Medicaid Services. 2007i (March). Medicare learning network, payment system fact sheet series. Inpatient rehabilitation facility prospective payment system. Available online from http://www.cms.hhs.gov/MLNProducts/downloads/IRFPPSFactSheet.pdf.

Centers for Medicare & Medicaid Services. 2007j (June 8). Inpatient rehabilitation facility PPS and the 75 percent rule. Available online from http://www.cms.hhs.gov/InpatientRehabFacPPS/Downloads/IRF_PPS_75_percent_Rule_060807.pdf.

Centers for Medicare & Medicaid Services. 2007k (May 4). Medicare program; Inpatient psychiatric facilities prospective payment system. Payment update for rate year beginning July 1, 2007 (RY 2008). *Federal Register* 72(86):25602–25673. Available online from http://www.cms.hhs.gov/quarterlyproviderupdates/downloads/cms1479n.pdf.

Centers for Medicare & Medicaid Services. 2007k (Aug. 1) Final Changes to the Hospital Inpatient Prospective Payment System, Final Rule. *Federal Register,* page 291

Centers for Medicare & Medicaid Services. 2006a (Nov. 3). Manual System: Pub 100-04, Medicare Claims Processing. Transmittal 1104, Change Request 5072. Available online from http://www.cms.hhs.gov/transmittals/downloads/R1104CP.pdf.

Centers for Medicare & Medicaid Services. 2006b (Oct. 27). Long Term Care Hospital PPS Overview. Available online from http://www.cms.hhs.gov/LongTermCareHospitalPPS/01_overview.asp.

Centers for Medicare & Medicaid Services. 2004a (June). Long-term care hospital prospective payment system news. Available online from http://www.cms.hhs.gov/LongTermCareHospitalPPS/Downloads/ltch_factsheet_fr.pdf.

Centers for Medicare & Medicaid Services. 2004b (April 1). Inpatient rehabilitation facility-patient assessment instrument training manual. Available online from http://www.cms.hhs.gov/InpatientRehabFacPPS/downloads/irfpaimanual040104.pdf.

Centers for Medicare and Medicaid Services (CMS). n.d.a. Updates and Revisions to ICD-9-CM Procedure Codes (Addendum), Volume 3. Available online from http://www.cms.hhs.gov/ICD9ProviderDiagnosticCodes/04_addendum.asp.

Centers for Medicare and Medicaid Services (CMS). n.d.b. Recovery audit contractor overview. Available online from http://www.cms.hhs.gov/RAC/.

Channel. 2008. *Educational Annotation of ICD-9-CM*. Reno, NV: Channel Publishing.

Department of Veterans Affairs. 2007 (Jan. 17). Health administration center. Available online from http://www.va.gov/hac/aboutus/programs/champva.asp.

Garrett, Gail. 2007. *Present on Admission*. Chicago: AHIMA.

HCA Management Services. 1995–2004. Policies and procedures. Available online from http://ec.hcahealthcare.com/CustomPage.asp?guidCustomContentID={A66C8906-BD78-4B3C-8D88-F4107A1E04CC}.

Health and Human Services. 2000 (October 5). OIG compliance plan. *Federal Register* 65(194):59434–59452. Available online from http://www.oig.hhs.gov/authorities/docs/physician.pdf.

Health and Human Services. 1985 (July 31). Uniform Hospital Discharge Data Set. *Federal Register* 50(147): 31038–40.

Health Insurance Association of America. 1995. *Managed Care: Integrating the Delivery and Financing of Health Care.* Washington, DC: America's Health Insurance Plans.

Homan, Cheryl. 2007. Functions of the health record. Chapter 2 in *Health Information Technology: An Applied Approach, 2nd ed.,* Merida Johns, editor. Chicago: AHIMA.

Hyde, Linda A., and Carol Spencer. 2008. *Analyzing the Financial Impact of MS-DRGs.* Chicago: AHIMA.

Ingenix. 2007 (Oct. 8). *Top 200 Coding Hospitals,* 4th annual edition. Eden Prairie, MN: Ingenix.

Jonas, Steven. 1998. *An Introduction to the U.S. Health Care System,* 4th ed. New York: Springer-Verlag.

Kaiser Permanente. n.d. Available online from http://newsmedia.kaiserpermanente.org/kpweb/historykp/ entrypage.do.

Kennedy, James. 2008. *Severity DRGs and Reimbursement: An MS-DRG Primer.* Chicago: AHIMA.

Medicare Payment Advisory Committee. 2005. Report to the Congress: Medicare payment policy. Washington, DC: MEDPAC. Available online from http://www.medpac.gov/documents/Mar05_EntireReport.pdf.

Monsees, Miller, Mayer, Presley & Amick. 2008. Available online from http://www.mmmpalaw.com/CM/ Articles/articles33.asp.

National Center for Health Statistics. 2007 (Sept. 6). *ICD-9-CM Official Guidelines for Coding and Reporting.* Available online from http://www.cdc.gov/nchs/datawh/ftpserv/ftpicd9/icdguide07.pdf.

National Committee on Vital and Health Statistics. 1996 (August). Core health data elements. Available online from http://ncvhs.hhs.gov/ncvhsr1.htm.

Newberry, Deb, and Gary Floss. 2003 (October). Six Sigma: Debunking the myths and delivering the goods. *Proceedings of the 75th Annual Convention and Exhibit: October 18–23* (Minneapolis, MN). Chicago: AHIMA.

Office of the Inspector General. 2005 (Jan. 31). Supplemental Compliance Program Guidance for Hospitals. *Federal Register* 70(19):4858–4876. Available online from http://oig.hhs.gov/fraud/docs/complianceguidance/ 012705HospSupplementalGuidance.pdf.

Office of the Inspector General. 1998 (Feb. 23). Publication of the OIG Compliance Program Guidance for Hospitals. *Federal Register,* 63(35):8987–8998. Available online from http://oig.hhs.gov/authorities/docs/cpghosp.pdf.

Office of the Inspector General. n.d. Work plan. Available online from http://oig.hhs.gov/publications/ workplan.html#1.

Prophet, Sue. 2001 (October). Practice brief: Developing a physician query process. *Journal of American Health Information Management Association* 72(9):88I–M.

QSource. 2005. Hospital payment monitoring program resources. Available online from http://www.qsource.org/ workbook.htm.

Quality Net. n.d. Reporting hospital quality data for annual payment update. Available online from http://www. qualitynet.org/dcs/ContentServer?cid=1138115987129&pagename=QnetPublic%2FPage%2FQnetTier2&c=Page.

Schraffenberger, Lou Ann, and Lynn Kuehn. 2007. *Effective Management of Coding Services: The Clinical Coding Manager's Handbook,* 3rd ed. Chicago: AHIMA.

Scott, Karen S. 2008. *Medical Coding for Non-Coders: Understanding Coding and Reimbursement for Today's Healthcare Industry.* Chicago: AHIMA.

Southeast Tennessee Legal Services n.d. Available online from http://www.selegal.org/glossary.htm.

Teslow, Mary Spivey. 2007. Health data concepts. Chapter 4 in *Health Information: Management of a Strategic Resource, 3rd ed.,* Mervat Abdelhak, et al., editors. Philadelphia: Saunders.

University of Tennessee. 2007. Physical therapy program. Available online from http://www.utmem.edu/allied/physical_therapy_home.html.

University of Texas. 2008. M.D. Anderson Cancer Center glossary of terms. Available online from http://www.mdanderson.org/patients_public/about_cancer/display.cfm?id=FA16B7A4-739D-11D4-AEBD 00508BDCCE3A&method=displayFull.

Wilson, Donna D. 2008. *Benchmarking to Improve Coding Accuracy and Productivity*. Rose Dunn, editor. Chicago: AHIMA.

Index

A, B, C, D, E audits, 179

Abnormal findings, reporting, 76, 84

Accommodations, inpatient, 10–12

Acute care hospital
POA reporting in, 80
PPSs in inpatient, 23
short- versus long-term, 13

Acute diagnosis codes, 33

Admission, identifying circumstances of, 73–74

Admission orders, coding professional's review of, 78

Admitting physician, responsibilities of, 3

Advanced chronic illnesses, 32

All-patient diagnosis-related groups (AP-DRGs), 43

American Health Information Management Association (AHIMA)
Code of Ethics of, 62, 149–57
coding recommendations of, 73
in Cooperating Parties, 62
data quality management model of, 94–97
members of, 149
Practice Brief: Developing a Coding Compliance Policy Document of, 159–63
Practice Brief: Developing a Physician Query Process of, 165–73
Practice Brief: Managing and Improving Data Quality of, 181–85
recommendation for incorporating query form in medical record by, 78
Standards of Ethical Coding of, 163, 168
Vision 2006 of, 180

American Hospital Association (AHA) in Cooperating Parties, 62

Ancillary services, types of services included for inpatient treatments as, 7–10

Anesthetic risk, occurrence of, 68

Angina, reporting, 84

Attending physician
role in consultations by specialists of, 75–76

verification of principal diagnosis with, 78, 122

Audit approach
for claims, 117, 192–98
for coding, 117–23, 188–92, 196–98
selecting, 188–89

Audit form
classifying changes to claims using, 197
samples of, 201–12
signature and dating of, 198

Audit plan
for claims audit, items included in, 193
for coding audit, documenting review using, 190–91

Audit strategy, 187–88

Audit team for coding audit, members of, 119

Audit tools
follow-up after completion of use of, 198
preparation for use of, 197
recording record, claim review, and findings using, 197
use in claims or coding review of, 196–97

Auditing processes, health record, 115–23
automation in, 180
corrective action following, 198
issues considered in, 115
plan of action for establishing or updating, 115

Auditing topics, recommended, 121

Auditors, selection of
for claims audit, 193
for coding audit, 190

Audits
baseline measurement in, 187–88, 196
claims, 117, 192–98
coding, 117–23, 188–92, 196–98
compliance program, 104–5, 106, 187–99
definition of, 187
policies and procedures, 117
problem types revealed by, 179
types of, 116
using results of, 192

Bacteremia, 102
Balanced Budget Act of 1997 (BBA)
    IME multiplier modified under, 38
    IRF PPS mandates by, 49
    long-term acute care hospital PPS required by, 47
Balanced Budget Refinement Act (BBRA)
    IME multiplier modified under, 38
    IPF PPS mandated by, 54
Balanced Budget Refinement Act of 1999, long-term acute care hospital PPS required by, 47
Bariatric surgery, 4
Benchmarking utilization and billing patterns, 107
Benefits Improvement and Protection Act (BIPA)
    IME multiplier modified under, 38
    long-term acute care hospital PPS required by, 47
Best practices, MS-DRGs for benchmarking, 44
Billing department role in claims audit, 194

Capitation for reimbursing inpatient services, 15
Cardiology as medical service division, 4
Cardiothoracic surgery, 4
Case examples for assigning principal and secondary diagnoses, 87–89, 113–14
Case management services
    cost control using, 21
    for inpatients, 10
Case mix, APC, 194
Case-mix groups
    components of, 51
    HIPPS codes grouped into, 49
    not included in RICs, table of, 53
    relative weights and average LOS for, 51
Case-mix index
    audit outcome focus on, 191
    as crude indicator in claims audits, 194
    example of, 107
    of hospital, average DRG weight in, 43
    resources used for Medicare patients tracked by, 106
Case rates basis for reimbursement contract, 15
Centers for Medicare and Medicaid Services (CMS)
    in Cooperating Parties, 62
    core elements of PPS described by, 30
    criminal investigations for fraud and abuse by, 104
    grouper program established by, 30
    QIO contracts with, 108
    services of long-term acute care hospitals described by, 13
    value-based purchasing strategy of, 20
Charge description master (CDM)
    charge line items generated from, 176–77
    claims audits including codes dropped in, 192

claims audits including individuals from departments using, 194
    ongoing review of, 184
Chronic illnesses, length of stay and, 32
Circumstances of admission, determining, 73–74. See also Present on admission (POA) diagnoses
Civilian Health and Medical Program of the Department of Veterans Affairs (CHAMPVA), 27
Claim accuracy, potential risk with, 117
Claim denials
    appealing inappropriate, 108
    monitoring, 108
    procedure for processing, 162
Claim re-billing
    cost of, 176
    pattern of, 197
Claims data profile of facility, software to develop, 192
Claims error rates, 182
Claims monitoring following coding and DRG revisions, 108
Clinical coding specialist (CCS), resources for, 69
Clinical data specialists, HIM, 183
Clinical documentation
    falsification of, 185
    as form of data collection, 177
    impact on healthcare industry revenues of, 61
Clinical documentation improvement program (CDIP), 79
Clinical documentation specialists (CDSs), 79
Clinical value compass data quality methodology, 97–98
CMS IRF-PAI Instruction Manual, 52
Coagulation disorders, RAC coding changes for, 102, 103
Code assignment
    correction of inaccurate, procedures for, 161
    description in coding compliance plan of parties responsible for, 160
    review of, in coding audit, 188
Code method in coding audits, 118–19
Code of Ethics (AHIMA), 62, 149–57
    applications of, 151
    interpretation of, 152–57
    purpose of, 150
    2004, 151–52
    use of, 150–51
    violation of, 150–51
Coder-to-coder peer review, 190
Coding accuracy, 166, 182
    coding audit study of, 188–92
    development of indicators for, 194
Coding and billing patterns, internal benchmarking of, 107
Coding audit. See Audits
Coding Audit Review Sheet, sample blank, 207–9

Coding Audit Summary form, sample blank, 205–6

Coding Clinic for ICD-9-CM
bleeding disorders resulting from Coumadin therapy in, 103
coder access to, 69
controversial issues identified in, 121
guidelines for coding pneumonia in, 109
official coding advice published in, 183
policies and procedures for each facility complying with usage in, 64
quarterly publication by AMA of, 63
septicemia in, 111

Coding compliance, 101–14

Coding compliance plan, components of and examples for, 159–63

Coding compliance policy document, developing, 159–63

Coding Compliance Review—Inpatient Summary form, sample blank, 210–12

Coding, DRG assignment and, 73–89

Coding error
education addressed to, 123
revised, added, or deleted code as, 118–19

Coding for inpatient services, 59–89
diagnostic and procedural, 61–72

Coding policies, 64–68
in coding compliance plan, 159
development of institutional, 64

Coding practices, evaluating internal, 106

Coding problem areas targeted by OIG, 109–12

Coding professionals
availability of documentation at time of coding by, 108
best practices adopted by, 183
data quality recommendations for, 183–85
decisions of, 73
dialogue between clinicians and, 168, 183
expectations and goals for, 167–68
health record review sequence used by, 77–78
internal auditors working with, 193
physician query by, 77–79

Coding professionals, professional ethics of, Code of Ethics of AHIMA detailing, 62, 149–57

Coding, relationship of documentation to, 166

Coding resources, identifying, 161

Coding review, retrospective, 189. *See also* Audits

Coding rules and guidelines, 62–64

Communication component of compliance plans, 106

Comorbidities
in IPF PPS, 55
in IRF PPS, 52
UDHHS definition of, 32, 66

Comparative data used in claims audit reports, 194–95

Compliance audit form, sample blank, 203–4

Compliance audit process, developing effective, 187–99

Compliance Coding Review Daily Worksheet, sample blank, 201

Compliance issues, corrective action and follow-up to correct, 106–7

Compliance officer, designation of, 106

Compliance program
auditing of, 104–5, 106
communication in, 106
components of, 105–8
key elements of effective, 104–5
key focus of, 180
OIG guidance for, 104
policies and procedures for, 105
training and education for, 106

Compliance Program Guidance (CPG) for hospitals, government, 106

Complication
checking daily documentation for development of, 77
definition by UHDDS of, 31–32, 65
described in progress notations, 65–66
identification of potential, 75

Complication or comorbidity (CC)
definition of, 31
exclusion list for Medicare of, 33–34
inclusion of, review of physician documentation for, 190
as middle level of severity for MS-DRGs, 42
secondary diagnosis as, 31

Complication or comorbidity (CC) list
major CC list versus, 32
revised in developing severity levels for MS-DRGs, 42

Comprehensive error rate testing (CERT) process, 182

Congestive heart failure (CHF), reporting, 84–85

Consolidated Omnibus budget Reconciliation Act of 1986 (COBRA)
disproportionate-share hospitals adjustment enacted by, 37
insurance coverage under, 28

Consultants, process improvement guidelines provided by, 180

Consultation reports, coding professional's review of, 78

Consultations by specialists, 75–76

Continuing education and training, completing, 184

Cooperating parties
for maintaining and updating ICD-9-CM, 62
primary role for *Coding Clinic* of, 63, 64

Coronary care unit, inpatients in, 11

Cosmetic surgery as type of plastic surgery, 4

Cost control methods, 20–21

CPT Assistant, coding advice published in, 183

Critical access hospital (CAH), 12, 13

Critical care unit (CCU), inpatients in, 11
per diem method of reimbursement for, 15–16

Cultures of body fluids, reviewing results of, 76

Daily documentation in health record, 77
Data accessibility, factors affecting, 95
Data accuracy, 94–95, 167, 168, 181
Data collection
    areas in hospital for, 176–77
    improving, 178–79
Data comparisons, 179
Data comprehensiveness for health records, 95
Data consistency, reliable data for, 95–96
Data currency, 96
Data definition, 96
Data dictionary, 177, 179
Data granularity, 96
Data integrity studies by OIG, 180
Data interpretation, 179
Data monitoring, 177–78
Data precision, 96–97
Data quality, 93–99
    approaches to controlling, 97–99
    definition of, 175
    impact on healthcare and HIM of, 175–80
    importance of, 176
    improvement of, 178–79
    managing and improving, 181–85
    mandates for, 181
    repetitive problems in, 179
    reporting root causes of concerns about, 183
Data quality cycle, 180
Data quality evaluation, critical elements in, 93
Data quality evaluation indicators identified for inpatients in coding audit, 122–23
Data quality evaluation process, role of coding managers in, 93
Data quality management and improvement initiatives, program actions of, 182–83
Data quality management model (AHIMA)
    quality management domains in, 94
    required characteristics of high-quality data in, 94–97
Data quality review results, reporting, 182
Data relevancy, 97
Databases
    challenges of maintaining accurate and meaningful, 181
    clinical, evaluation of, 182
    decisions regarding uses of, 179
Débridement fascia/muscle, 103
Deficit Reduction Act (DRA) requirements for hospital-acquired conditions, 81
Denial spreadsheet for denied and returned claims, example of, 108
Department of Health and Human Services (HHS) transaction and coding standards regulations, 63
Department of Veterans Affairs statistics for VA healthcare system, 12–13
Diagnoses
    additional, complications as, 65
    cause of symptom or sign stated in, 82
    frequently overlooked, 85–86

    guidelines for coding multiple, 81–82
    inconsistencies among types of, 96
    invalid, MCE detection of, 70
    unusual, process for coding, 161
Diagnosis-related group (DRG) assignment
    coding and, 73–89
    factors influencing, 34
    principal diagnosis as usually determining, 67
    review in claims audits of, 195
    severity of illness not always reflected in, 42
    validation studies of, 111
    variables in, 31–32
Diagnosis-related groups (DRGs)
    claims monitoring following updates to, 108
    comparison between MS-DRGs and, 44
    definition of, 29
    fiscal intermediary using grouper for assigning, 30
    for inpatient psychiatric PPS, 54, 55
    modifications in. See All-patient diagnosis-related groups (AP-DRGs)
    modified for TRICARE for Life medical coverage, 26
    relative weights of, 35–44
    review of problematic, 189
    targeted by RACs, 101–3
Discharge status codes, 71–72, 122
Discharge summary, post-discharge documentation included in, 171
Discharges, transfers versus, 40
Disease process, coding conditions that are and are not integral part of, 84
Disproportionate-share hospitals, inpatient PPS reimbursement adjusted for, 36–37
Documentation completeness, monitoring, 21
Documentation disputes with physicians, resolving, 162
Documentation guidelines for physician queries, 79
Documentation, health record
    adding, protocols for, 160
    patterns of poor, 172
    principles of, 165
    relationship of coding to, 166
    requirements of, rules for, 167
Documentation improvement program, 184
Documentation requirements for compliance plans, 108
Duplicate diagnosis error, 70
Durable medical equipment (DME), Medicare Part B to reimburse, 24

E codes, clarification of appropriate use of, 161
Electroconvulsive therapy (ECT), additional payment to IPF PPS for, 55
Emergency department record, coding professional's review of, 74
Emergency Medical Treatment and Labor Act (EMTALA), 116

Employers, group medical insurance plans sponsored by, 27
Encoders, reliance on, 162
Erroneous claims, 103
  costs of rebilling, 176
Error rate, coding, 191
Errors in data, analysis of, 178, 182
Ethics of health information coding professionals
  challenges to, 181, 182–83
  Code of Ethics (AHIMA) for, 62, 149–57
  Standards of Ethical Coding (AHIMA) for, 163, 168

Facility base rate in Medicare inpatient PPS reimbursement, 39
Facility- or practice-specific coding guidelines, 64, 183
Federal Civil False Claims Act (FCA), 104
Federal Register
  relative weights for DRGs published annually in, 35
  revisions to ICD-9-CM published in, 63
Fee-based services, reimbursement of, 16–17
Fee-for-service method for reimbursing inpatient services, 15
  Medicare originally based on, 22
  traditional, comparison of managed care and, table of, 17
  used commonly prior to managed care era, 15, 16
Fee schedules for reimbursement of physician and ancillary services, 16
Final diagnostic statement, diagnoses not listed in, 84, 190
Financial services, MS-DRGs used in, 44
First Look Analysis Tool for Hospital Outlier Monitoring (FATHOM), 182
Fiscal intermediary (FI), hospital inpatient claims for CMS processed by, 30
Focused coding reviews, 121–22
For-profit hospitals, 12
Forms control, 177
Fraud and abuse, 103–5
  claims of, statute of limitations for, 104
  data patterns indicating, 182
  definition of, 103
  legislation to combat, 69
  OIG monitoring system for, 180
Frequently overlooked diagnoses, list of, 85–86
Frequently overlooked procedures, list of, 86–87
Functional independence measures–functional related groups (FIM-FRGs), 49

Gastroenterology, specialty services of, 4
Graduate medical education (GME) program, additional Medicare payments for IME costs for, 38
Group medical insurance plans, commercial and nonprofit, 27–28
Group model HMO, 18
  Kaiser Permanente as example of, 19

Grouper software in assigning DRGs
  for IPPS, 30
  for LTCH PPS, 48

Health information management (HIM) professional. *See also* Coding professional
  actions prohibited for, 184–85
  as advocate for profession, 156
  ethical obligations of, 149, 183. *See also* Ethics of health information coding professionals
  future of, 180, 183
  professional values of, 149–50, 167
  responsibilities for accuracy of coded data as shared with others by, 181
  UR performed by, 21
Health Insurance Portability and Accountability Act of 1996 (HIPAA)
  electronic transaction standards of, modifications to, 183
  healthcare coverage as portable under, 28
  official code sets under, 63
  Privacy rule compliance under, 116
  Security rule compliance under, 116
  transactions standards of, 63
Health insurance prospective payment system (HIPPS) codes, grouping into case-mix groups of, 49
Health maintenance organizations (HMOs)
  as type of MCO, 17
  types of, 17–19
Health record
  auditing processes for, 115–23
  coding process using entire, 183
  completion deadline for, 166
  cost control using retrospective reviews of, 21
  data elements generally required for, 95
  incomplete, assigning codes to, 185
  inconsistencies in, 96
  sections of, 74–77
  sequence for review of, suggested, 77–78
  size of, increasing, 178
  support for clinical codes reported in, 184
  timely entries to, 165–66
Health record review, Joint Commission requirements for, 166
History and physical examination
  coding professional's review of, 78
  in initial database of health record, 75
Home healthcare settings, PPS in, 23
Hospital Payment Monitoring Program (HPMP), 109
  FATHOM developed under, 182
  method and structure for evaluating coding and reimbursement resulting from, 116
Hospital performance statistics, comparison by benchmarking of, 107
Hospital reimbursement program of Blue Cross and Blue Shield, 27
Hospital-specific relative value method adjustment for LTCH PPS, 49
Hospitals, types of, 12–13
  PPSs in various, 23

ICD-9-CM Coordination and Maintenance
　　Committee, 63
ICD-9-CM Official Guidelines for Coding
　　and Reporting, 64
　　applying, case examples for, 87–89
　　code assignment rules of, 64
　　coding abnormal findings described in, 76
　　in coding compliance plan, 159
　　developed by Cooperating Parties, 63
　　for LTCH PPS coding guidance, 48
　　as official standard for coding diagnoses
　　　　and procedures under HIPAA, 63
　　training coding audit team in use of, 119
Indemnity insurance plans, 22
Independent model HMO, 18
Indicators, defining audit
　　for claims audit, 194, 195–96
　　for coding audit, 191–92
Indirect medical education (IME) costs of
　　teaching hospitals, inpatient PPS
　　adjustment for, 38
Individual medical insurance, 27
Inpatient coding quality measures, 117–18
Inpatient Prospective Payment System (IPPS),
　　acute care, 29–45
　　adjustments to standard reimbursement to,
　　　　35–43
　　development of, 30–31
　　DRGs in. See Diagnosis-related groups
　　　　(DRGs)
　　Final Rule of, 80–81
　　hospitals exempt from, 39–40
　　ICD-9-CM codes as basis for updated
　　　　DRGs and grouper software used by
　　　　LTCH PPS and, 30
　　reimbursement to, disproportionate-share
　　　　hospitals receiving additional, 36–37
　　shared payments for transfers under, 40
　　updates to, 41–42
Inpatient psychiatric facilities PPS (IPF PPS),
　　vii, 23
　　comorbidity groupings in, 55–56
　　DRGs for, table of, 55
　　payment adjustments for, 54–57
Inpatient psychiatric facility, PPS in, vii, 23,
　　54–57
Inpatient rehabilitation facilities (IRFs)
　　percentage rate for patient conditions
　　　　counting in, 54
　　PPS in, vii, 23, 49–54
　　preadmission screening and Medicare
　　　　coverage for, 5
　　qualifying as, 52–54
Inpatient rehabilitation facility patient
　　assessment instrument (IRF PAI), 49, 52
Inpatient Rehabilitation Validation and Entry
　　(IRVEN) software, 49
Inpatient Review Variations by Coder form,
　　sample blank, 202
Inpatient services
　　introduction to, 3–13
　　process for coding and reimbursement of,
　　　　91–123
　　reimbursement for, 1–57

Inpatients, definition of, 3
Intensive care unit (ICU), inpatients in, 11
Internal medicine as medical service division, 4
International Classification of Diseases,
　　9th Revision, Clinical Modification
　　(ICD-9-CM) codebook
　　Alphabetic Index of, 73
　　as basis for updated DRGs and grouper
　　　　software used by IPPS and LTCH PPS,
　　　　30, 41
　　coder access to, 69
　　coding experience with, vii
　　Cooperating Parties for maintaining and
　　　　updating, 62
　　DRGs for complete range of diagnoses
　　　　in, 30
International Classification of Diseases,
　　9th Revision, Clinical Modification
　　(ICD-9-CM) codes
　　assignment of, 73
　　modifications to, 63
　　validation by MCE of, 69
Interrupted stays, payments for
　　in IPF PPS, 55, 57
　　in LTC PPS, 48
Invalid coding entries, MCE to detect, 69–72

Joint Commission
　　coding audit sample recommendations of,
　　　　120
　　medical record standards of, 165–66, 181
Joint replacements, 103

Labor and non-labor-related costs for DRG
　　amount, 35–36
Laboratory services for inpatients, 7–8
Length of stay (LOS)
　　acute conditions affecting, 33
　　geometric and arithmetic mean, 40, 41
Local Coverage Determinations (LCDs), 23
Local Medical Review Policies (LMRPs), 23
Long-term acute care hospitals, Medicare
　　definition of, 13
Long-term care facilities, interrupted stays
　　in, 48
Long-term care hospital PPS (LTCH PPS),
　　vii, 23, 47–49
　　ICD-9-CM codes as basis for updated
　　　　DRGs and grouper software used by
　　　　IPPS and, 30
　　major elements of, 48–49
　　patient classification system using
　　　　DRG-type groupings in, 48
　　rate of payment for, 48–49
　　transition period to phase in, 49

Major CC list, CC list versus, 32
Major complication or comorbidity (MCC) as
　　highest severity level for CCs, 42–43
Major diagnostic categories (MDCs), multiple
　　DRGs contained in, 34–35
Major medical coverage of Blue Cross and
　　Blue Shield, 27

Managed care organizations (MCOs) as capitated payment plans, 17
Managed care payment systems
  characteristics of, 17
  fee-for-service traditional insurance plans contrasted with, 16–17
Master patient index (MPI), 176
  improving data in, 178–79
Medicaid billing, risk areas in, 116
Medicaid Eligibility Summary, 25
Medicaid program, 25
Medical necessity
  assessed during preadmission review, 20
  for private rooms of inpatients, 10–11
Medical record. *See* Health record
Medical services
  definition of, 4
  divisions of, 4
Medical social services for inpatients, 10
Medicare billing, risk areas in, 116
Medicare Code Editor (MCE) software, types of errors detected by, 69–72
Medicare Conditions of Participation, health record requirements of, 166, 181
Medicare-dependent rural hospitals (MDHs), DRG rate formula higher for, 39
Medicare DRG Handbook, The, code audits using, 117
Medicare Modernization Act (MMA), Medicare payment updates under, 109
Medicare programs
  complication or comorbidity exclusion list by, 33–34
  Medicare Advantage-Prescription Drug (MA-PD), 25
  original design of, 21
  overpayments to, RAC analysis of, 101–2
  Part A inpatient hospitalization, 24
  Part B physician and outpatient services, DME and supplies, 24
  Part C (Medicare Advantage), 24
  Part D Medicare Prescription Drug Plan, 24–25
  Pay for Performance (P4P) initiative of, 20
  postacute care transfer policy of, 34, 40, 41
  prospective payments systems of. *See* Prospective payment systems (PPSs), Medicare
Medicare Provider Analysis and Review (MEDPAR) file, 195
  Medicare DRG Handbook compiled from, 117
  RAC analysis of, 102
Medicare reimbursement for inpatients, MS-DRGs for, 16
Medicare severity adjusted diagnosis related groups (MS-DRGs)
  base groups of, 43
  case-mix index as average weight of, 43
  comparisons between DRGs and, 44
  division into subgroups of, 43
  DRG system revamped to create, 42, 47
  error, 43
  groupings and weights of, to determine payment, table of, 26

list of, 50
  for Medicare inpatient reimbursement, 16, 20, 29, 30
  process of, diagram of, 34
  relative weights of, 35, 41
  uses of, 43–45
  for utilization review, 43
Medicare Severity-adjusted Long-term Care Hospital Diagnosis Related Groups (MS-LTC-DRGs)
  grouping of patient stays into, 47
  relative weights of, 48
Military healthcare programs, 25–27
Most significant diagnoses, 67

National Center for Health Statistics (NCHS) in Cooperating Parties, 62
National Committee on Vital and Health Statistics (NCVHS), classifications and terminology for inpatient PPS prescribed by, 30
National coverage determinations (NCDs), 23
National Uniform Billing Committee (NUBC), uniform billing forms developed by, 64
Neonatal intensive care unit (NICU), inpatients in, 11
Network model HMO, 18
Neurology, specialty services of, 4
Neurosurgery, 5
New procedures or unusual diagnoses, procedure for coding, 161
New technology, facility payment rate adjusted by Medicare for use of, 38–39
Nonspecific or noncovered operating room procedures, MCE detection of, 71
Not-for-profit hospitals, 12
Nursery unit, newborns in, 12
Nursing professional, UR performed by, 21
Nursing services for inpatients, 7

Obstetrics/gynecology as medical service division, 4
Occupational mix adjustment affecting wages in facility payment rate, 35–36
Occupational therapy services for inpatients, 8–9
Office of the Inspector General (OIG)
  coding and payment problem areas targeted by, 109–12
  Compliance Program Guidance for Hospitals of, 172
  federal audits by, 104
  fraud and abuse monitoring system of, 180, 197
  guidance for compliance programs by, 104–5
  Office of Audit Services Statistical Sampling Software of, 191
  study of DRG assignment and coding accuracy, 67
  test of upcoding software by, 193
  2005 Supplemental Compliance Program Guidance for Hospitals of, 116

Official Authorized Addendum to the ICD-9-CM, revisions published in, 63
Official Coding Guidelines for ICD-9-CM. *See* ICD-9-CM Official Guidelines for Coding and Reporting
Open-biopsy check by MCE, 71
Operation Restore Trust, 104
Optional codes gathered for statistical purposes, 161
Oral and maxillofacial surgery, 5
Orthopedics, specialty services of, 4
Other diagnoses
    definition of, 83
    guidelines for designating and reporting, 83–87
    UHDDS definition of, 65
Outliers
    additional payments by IPF PPS for, 57
    additional payments by IPPS for, 30, 39
    short-stay, 48
Outpatient hospitals, PPSs in, 23
Outpatient records, claims audit of, 197

Patient assessment instrument (PAI) for rehabilitation hospital inpatients, 49, 52
Patients, risk areas for inappropriate incentives for, 116
Pay for performance (P4P) initiatives
    CMS, for hospital-acquired conditions, 80–81
    development of, 20
Payer-specific reporting requirements, 160–61
Payers, common types of healthcare, 21–28
Payment Error Prevention Program (PEPP), 109, 116, 187
Payment methods for inpatient services, 15–16
Payments to reduce or limit services, risk with, 116
Pediatrics as medical service division, 4
Peer review organizations (PROs), 187
Per diem method of reimbursement, 15–16
    for IPF PPS, 54
Per resident amount (PRA) for direct medical education costs, 38
Physical therapy, definition of, 8
Physical therapy services for inpatients, 8
Physician advisor for coding audits, 190
Physician documentation
    baseline review in coding audit of, 188–90
    clarification of, 108
    codes not assigned without, 163
    coding professional's review of, 77–78
    as cornerstone of accurate coding, 166, 182
    education by healthcare team to improve, 183
    expectations about, 167
    in principal diagnosis selection, 74
    for query, 78
Physician liaison, appropriate use of, 169
Physician offices, PPSs for services in, 23

Physician orders
    in daily documentation section of health record, 77
    data collection beginning with, 176
Physician participation in active psychiatric treatment, 7
Physician queries
    for cause and effect relationship, 77
    clinical criteria for valid, 170
    concurrent, 169
    documenting response to, 170–71
    goal of, 168
    proper use of, 168–71, 184
    response to, 123
    sample blank, 173
    situations not warranting, 170
Physician query process
    for condition identified but not documented, 75
    developing, 165–73
    failure to use, 185
    importance of, 111
    policy for, 78
Physician self-referral law, 116
Physician services, reimbursement of
    Medicare Part B for, 24
    in PPO network, 19
Plan of psychiatric treatment recorded in accordance with Medicare Conditions of Participation for Hospitals, 6
Plastic surgery, 4
Pneumonias
    coding problem areas with, 109
    comparison of patients with complex compared to community acquired, 122
Point-of-service (POS) plan
    out-of-network services allowed in, 19
    as type of MCO, 17
Postacute care payment policy, Medicare, 34, 40, 41
Preadmission review
    cost control using, 20–21
    insurance plans requiring, 22
Preferred payment plan of Blue Cross and Blue Shield, 27
Preferred provider organizations (PPOs)
    elements of services of, 19
    as type of MCO, 17
Prescription drug plan (PDP), Medicare, 24
Present on admission (POA) diagnoses, 79–81
Principal diagnosis
    coding professional's confirmation of, 78
    definition in UHDDS of, 31, 65, 122, 197
    diagnostic tests to justify, 76
    E code not used as, 70
    manifestation code as, as error, 70
    nonspecific, 70
    principal procedure as one most related to, 68–69
    selection of, 67, 197
    steps in record review to determine, 73, 77–78
    unacceptable, 70

Principal inpatient diagnostic cost group (PIP-DCG) algorithm, 24
Principal procedure, selecting, 68–69
Procedural risk of procedures, 67–68
Procedures, frequently overlooked, 86–87
Processes for coding and reimbursement of inpatient services, 91–123
Professional values of HIM professionals, 149–50, 167
Progress notes
    coder review of, 76, 78
    in daily documentation, 77
    physician's recordings and conclusions in, 74
    query form for, sample blank, 173
Prospective payment systems (PPSs), Medicare
    characteristics of, 22–23
    core elements in, 30
    fee-for-service system replaced by, 22
    home healthcare (HH-PPS), 23
    inpatient (IPPS), vii, 23, 29–45
    inpatient psychiatric facility (IPF-PPS), vii, 23, 54–57
    inpatient rehabilitation facilities (IRF-PPS), vii, 23, 49–54
    long-term care (LTCH-PPS), vii, 23, 47–49
    modified by other payers, 20
    need for managing coded data effectively in, 61
    outpatient hospital (OPPS), 23
    reimbursement in, 19–20
    settings for, healthcare, 23
    stop-loss provision for, 54
Psychiatric services
    definition of, 6
    Medicare reimbursement criteria for, 6–7
Pulmonary medicine, specialty services of, 4

Quality data. See Data quality
Quality data requirements of Medicare Modernization Act, 109
Quality improvement organizations (QIOs)
    coding workbook by, 112
    questionable admissions reviewed by, 70
    resources on compliance programs provided by, 116
Quality measures, inpatient coding, 117–18
Quality of care, risk areas with, 116
Query form for physician queries, 78–79
    filed in medical record, obtaining advice for, 171
    format of, 169–70
    judicious use of, 168
    sample blank, 173
Query practice, periodic review of, 171–72
Query response, documenting, 170–71
Questionable admission, MCE detection of, 70

Radiology services for inpatients, 7
Rebilling claims
    cost of, 176
    pattern of, 197

Reconstructive surgery as type of plastic surgery, 4
Record method in coding audit, 118
Recovery audit contractors (RACs), 101–3
    initial targets of, 101–2
    top DRGs for, 102–3
Recuperative care unit, inpatients in, 12
Rehabilitation impairment categories (RICs) in IRF PPS, 51
    list of, 51
Rehabilitation services, 5–6
Reimbursement
    coding errors affecting, audit study of, 191
    discharge status for transfer patients affecting, 40
    for inpatient services, 1–57
    maximizing, coding for, 162
Reimbursement methodologies for inpatient services, 15–28
    arrangements made by insurance carriers using, 16–20
    cost control methods in, 20–28
    payment methods for, 15–20
Reimbursement system for government programs, transition in, 94
Requirements for Hospital Reporting of Quality Data for Annual Payment Update, 109
Resource tools, ongoing review of, 184
Respiratory therapy services for inpatients, 9
Results, audit
    for coding audit, presenting, 123
    compiling, 192, 195–96
    using, 192, 196
Retrospective review of health record, cost control using, 21
Risks of medical care
    areas of, 116
    described in coding compliance plan, 161
    OIG Workplan identification of, 189
    types of, 67–68

Sample size for coding audit, 119–20
Scope of Work (SOW), QIO, 108
Secondary diagnosis
    additional diagnosis as, 75
    as CC, 31–34
    coding, 78
    coding professional's verification of, 78
    diagnostic tests to support coding of, 76
    LOS affected by, 77
    medications associated with, 75
    UHDDS definition of, 31
Secondary payers, MCE alert for, 71
Sepsis
    review of patients with UTI versus, 122
    severe, 110, 111
    treatment of, 112
Septic shock, 110, 112
Septicemia
    coding problem areas with, 110–12
    RAC coding changes for, 102–3
Severe sepsis, 110, 111

Short-term acute care hospitals, 13
Significant procedures, reporting all, 67
Six Sigma approach to data quality, 97
Skilled nursing unit
    per diem method of reimbursement for, 16
    PPSs in, 23
Social Security Act
    Medicaid as Title XIX of, 25
    PPS mandated by TEFRA amendments
      to, 29
Sole community hospitals (SCHs), DRG rate
    formula higher for, 39
Source document, collection of data in, 177
Special units, patient accommodations in,
    11–12
Specialized training, procedures involving,
    68–69
Speech therapy services for inpatients, 9–10
Staff model HMO, 18
Standards of Ethical Coding (AHIMA), 163,
    168
Surgery clearance, 76
Surgical hierarchy in MDC, 35
Surgical services, divisions based on body
    systems for, 4–5
Swing bed for either acute care or skilled
    care, 12
Symptoms, signs, and ill-defined conditions,
    coding, 82–83
Systemic inflammatory response syndrome
    (SIRS), 110

Tax Equity and Fiscal Responsibility Act
    (TEFRA), inpatient PPS mandated by,
    29
Teaching facilities, IPF PPS payment
    adjustment for, 54, 57
Teaching hospitals, inpatient PPS adjustment
    for indirect medical education (IME)
    costs of, 38
Therapeutic procedures, coder review in
    health record of, 76–77
Traditional healthcare insurance. *See* Fee-
    for-service method for reimbursing
    inpatient services

Training and education for compliance plan,
    106
Transplant surgery, 5
Trend analysis of claims audit results, 196
TRICARE medical coverage types for service
    members, 25–26

Uniform Bill-82 (UB-82), 64
Uniform Bill-04 (UB-04) form, 64, 177
Uniform Hospital Discharge Data Set
    (UHDDS)
    coding policy compliance with, 73
    definition of principal diagnosis in, 31, 65,
      122, 197
    definition of secondary diagnosis in, 31
    definitions and systemized terminology of,
      48, 64
    development of, 65
    links in facility's coding guidelines to, 163
    relationship to coding of, 65–68
    sequencing guidelines of, as prescribed by
      NCVHS for inpatient PPS, 30
    significant versus non-significant
      procedures for, 5
    UB-04 containing most items of, 177
Upcoding, software to detect, 193
Urinary tract infection (UTI), 102, 122
Urology, specialty services of, 4
Urosepsis, physician query for, 111
Utilization review (UR)
    cost control using, 21
    focus on atypical patients of, 29
    in managed care systems, rigorous, 17
    MS-DRGs used for, 43
    by PPOs, 19
    in PPS reimbursement systems, 22

Value-based purchasing (CMS), 20
Veterans hospitals, 12–13

Wage index of labor costs for PPS, 30
Wound débridement and skin graft, RAC
    coding changes for, 103